DR. SEBI KIDNEY FAILURE SOLUTION

THE MOST COMPLETE MANUAL TO NATURALLY TREAT CHRONIC KIDNEY DISEASE (CKD) AND STAY OFF DIALYSIS

By Serena Brown

Copyright © 2020 by Serena Brown - All rights reserved.

This document is geared towards providing exact and reliable information in regards to the topic and issue covered. The publication is sold with the idea that the publisher is not required to render an account officially permitted or otherwise qualified services. If advice is necessary, legal or professional, a practiced individual in the profession should be ordered.

In no way is it legal to reproduce, duplicate, or transmit any part of this document by either electronic means or in printed format. The recording of this publication is strictly prohibited, and any storage of this document is not allowed unless with written permission from the publisher. All rights reserved.

The information provided herein is stated to be truthful and consistent. In terms of inattention or otherwise, any liability, by any use or abuse of any policies, processes, or directions contained within is the recipient reader's solitary and utter responsibility. Under no circumstances will any reparation, damages, or monetary loss due to the information herein, either directly or indirectly

Disclaimer Notice: Please note the information contained within this document is for educational and entertainment purposes only. Every attempt has been made to provide accurate, up to date and reliable, complete information. No warranties of any kind are expressed or implied. Reader acknowledges that the author is not engaging in the rendering of legal, financial, medical, or professional advice. The content of this book has been derived from various sources. Please consult a licensed professional before attempting any techniques outlined in this book.

Table of Contents

INTRODUCTION 4

CHAPTER 1: KIDNEYS 6

CHAPTER 2: CHRONIC KIDNEY DISEASE (CKD) 15

CHAPTER 3: KIDNEY FAILURE 21

CHAPTER 4: CAUSES OF CKD 27

CHAPTER 5: SYMPTOMS OF CKD 29

CHAPTER 6: CORRELATION WITH OTHER DISEASES 31

CHAPTER 7: CONVENTIONAL TREATMENTS 35

CHAPTER 8: DR. SEBI AND KIDNEY'S HEALTH 38

CHAPTER 9: AVOIDING DIALYSIS 46

CHAPTER 10: DR. SEBI METHOD TO HEAL KIDNEYS 48

CHAPTER 11: SUPPLEMENTS 87

CONCLUSION 92

Introduction

Regarding your well-being and health, it's a smart thought to see your doctor as frequently as conceivable to ensure you don't run into preventable issues that you needn't get. The kidneys are your body's toxin channel (just like the liver), cleaning the blood of remote substances and toxins discharged from things like preservatives in food & other toxins.

Kidney disease is a growing health concern for many people and can often lead to chronic infections, impaired function, and in serious cases, renal failure. When kidneys fall below 25 % of their ability to filter and clear waste from the body, they are no longer able to continue without the support of dialysis or a complete transplant. While many causes may lead to various forms of kidney impairment, one of the best ways to prevent and treat renal failure is a healthy, sensible diet. This book will provide the necessary steps you can take to significantly improve your health and prognosis after a renal failure diagnosis and show you how to prevent further damage to your kidneys, whether your condition is in the beginning stages or more advanced. Learning how to manage your diet and choose the right foods for your kidneys and overall health is vital to improving your chances of enjoying a healthy and productive life.

According to the physician and dietitian's advice, people with chronic kidney disease should change their diet to reduce the impaired kidney's burden and prevent distress in fluid and electrolyte balance. There is no fixed diet for patients with chronic kidney disease. Each patient is given different nutritional recommendations depending on the clinical condition, renal failure stage, and other medical problems. It is also necessary to change the dietary recommendations for the same patient at different times.

Since kidneys are vital for the human body's proper functioning, you need to take good care of them. The first step for having healthy kidneys would be to incorporate all you have read about in this book. You should also make sure that these practices become a habit for you, and you will start to notice a positive change in your overall health!

Kidney failure has no treatment to reverse it, and it is essential to take a truly healthy diet that protects your body from any kind of health hazards associated with kidney disease. However, if you suffer from kidney failure or any other kidney disease, there is no reason to give up hope; with proper treatment and diet, the management you can live a healthy and long life.

All you have to do is start making healthy lifestyle choices, and it begins with healthy changes to your diet. The good news is that once you start your kidney treatment and maintain your ideal diet, its associated symptoms begin to go away.

Good dietary habits are known to keep kidney diseases at bay. It's time to make smart choices when it comes to food that you eat every day. An ideal renal diet is all about including wholesome foods and reducing the number of products, which contain high sodium, high phosphorous, and high potassium.

This book provides a comprehensive list of kidney-friend foods recommended by Dr. Sebi. People worldwide suffer from some kind of disease, but we all have to still keep on living even though it might be a little more difficult. Those who have renal disease can replenish vitamins and necessary nutrients by following a diet. People with mild complications may tweak their food slightly; however, those with end-stage renal disease must follow a doctor's strict diet.

When it comes to your health and well-being, it's a good idea to see the doctor as often as possible to make sure you don't run into any major problems. The kidneys are your body's drug reservoir (as is the liver), cleansing the blood of foreign substances and contaminants released by food-related preservatives and other toxins.

Chapter 1: Kidneys

Kidneys are two organs about your fist's size located near the bottom of your rib cage, on either side of the spine. Millions of tiny things called 'nephrons' in each kidney serve to filter the blood.

Kidney disease will attack these nephrons. The damage it causes might leave the kidneys unable to get rid of the waste. There are about 26 million people in the United States who are affected by kidney disease. That happens when the kidneys get damaged and aren't able to function properly. This damage might be caused by different long-term chronic conditions, high blood pressure, and diabetes. Kidney disease could cause other problems such as malnutrition, nerve damage, and weak bones.

If it gets worse with time, the kidneys might completely stop working altogether. That means that you might have to undergo dialysis to help the kidneys perform. Dialysis is a medical treatment where a machine purifies and filters the blood. This won't cure the disease, but it does help prolong life.

Understanding how a disease works is not as simple as telling someone that the letter B comes after A. We need first to recognize the functions of a kidney. That way, we might understand just how the disease affects the organ.

When they are functioning normally, kidneys are responsible for crucial jobs, such as:

- Clear out waste substances and materials from your blood

- Flush out excess water from your body

- Manage your blood pressure

- Encourage your bone marrow to produce red blood cells

- Restrict the amount of phosphorus and calcium absorbed and excreted

You might be surprised by some of the responsibilities above. Some people raise their eyebrows in surprise when they realize that our kidneys are responsible for stimulating our bone marrow to produce red blood cells, or RBCs. But that is how versatile our kidneys are.

The feature that interests us is the fact that our kidneys help in filtering blood. There are a million filtering units in the bean-shaped organs. In turn, these units, called nephrons, have a filter known as a glomerulus along with another component called "tubule". Those are some pretty complex terms but don't worry; I shall not drop a biology explanation.

To put it simply, a glomerulus is a modified blood vessel. Typically, your normal blood vessels transport blood throughout the body. The glomerulus, on the other hand, filters your blood to create urine. But once the urine has been produced, what happens to it? Are glomeruli going to do all the work of transporting them to your bladder?

That's where tubules come into play. These tiny structures take the waste materials from the glomerulus, look through them to see if any useful materials might have been included by accident, then passes on the useful materials back to the blood and urine to the pelvis. Think of this arrangement as a nightclub with two bouncers. The first bouncer is dealing with a large crowd outside. You might take advantage of that fact and sneak in, only to realize that a second guard is waiting for you, who has his job made easier because the first guard has whittled down the crowd to a manageable number. This time, you better be right about the age in your ID.

It's like your body created its version of the two-step verification process that you find when you try to open your bank account online or log into certain websites; fluids get 'verified' for good materials first by the glomerulus, then by tubules. But it is necessary because your body is trying to filter your blood properly.

How the Kidneys Work

Our kidneys are bean-shaped filters that work in teams. They have a very important job since they keep our bodies stable. They use signals from the body like blood pressure and sodium content to help keep us hydrated and our blood pressure stable.

If the kidneys don't function right, numerous problems could happen. When these toxins' filtration becomes slow, these harmful chemicals can build up and cause other body reactions like vomiting, nausea, and rashes. When the kidney's functions continue to decrease, its ability to get rid of water and release hormones that control blood pressure can also be affected. Symptoms such as high blood pressure or retaining water in your feet might happen. With time having reduced kidney function could cause long-term health problems such as osteoporosis or anemia.

The kidneys work hard, so we have to protect them. They can filter around 120 to 150 quarts of blood each day. This will create between 1 and 2 quarts of urine made up of excess fluid and waste products.

When Your Kidney Functions Get Kidnapped

According to the National Kidney Foundation, the two main causes of chronic kidney disease are high blood pressure and diabetes (National Kidney Foundation, n.d.). If you visit a doctor, health expert, or diet consultant, you will realize that one of the major ways to manage your blood pressure and prevent diabetes is a healthy diet. But more on that later.

As the blood pressure or diabetes levels get worse, so does the amount of waste build-up. The waste goes into your blood faster than the kidneys can filter them. At this point, your kidneys are like an overworked employee at a firm; there is so much work remaining, but only a small amount of time to get finished during a particular period. The kidneys begin to deteriorate over time. The filters start to leak, unable to hold on to the waste build-up anymore. Only a small percentage of the entire waste gets filtered properly, with the rest entering the bloodstream. For some, the time it takes for kidney failure might be months, while for others, the kidneys could worsen across a span of years. It all depends on numerous factors like diet, lifestyle choices, and even genetics.

Pretty soon, you might feel like your kidney functions have been kidnapped; they don't seem to be functioning well anymore, or they barely exist. But that is not the case. Think of the example of the overworked employee that we used earlier. At some point, the employee could collapse out of dehydration or exhaustion. Similarly, kidney disease causes the organs to fail, which causes numerous problems such as low energy, high exhaustion levels, sleep difficulties, poor appetite, swollen ankles and feet, and the need to urinate more often, especially at night.

Many people mistakenly believe the kidneys act as sponges, which is far from the truth. The kidneys do not absorb and hold onto waste and harmful compounds. Instead, the kidneys filter out these toxins so that they can be completely removed from the body. They do this with a complex system that consists of millions of nephrons, which are microscopic filters. Nephrons are comprised of two components, which are the glomerulus and the tubule. In order to cleanse the blood, the glomerulus strains it of the larger molecules from fluid and waste. After this pass through the glomerulus, they head to the tubule. As the blood travels through the tubule component of the nephrons, smaller molecules of waste are collected. Not only that, but the tubule also collects any minerals found within the blood and then transfers them back into the bloodstream. But how are these toxins removed from the kidneys and the body so that they don't stay stuck within your organs? When the kidneys filter water from your bloodstream, it combines the water with the filtered waste and toxins, allowing them to be carried to the bladder before being expelled from the body.

Some of the waste that the kidneys remove from your blood is excess acid produced in your blood to maintain healthy minerals and water levels. This acid affects the levels of many minerals, such as potassium, sodium, calcium, and phosphorus. When these minerals are out of balance, your body will be unable to function properly. As these minerals are electrolytes, they affect the maintenance and control of your muscles, nerves, tissues, and balance. Without the proper balance of these electrolytes, you can be in a rather dangerous situation.

Athletes are frequently aware of the importance of maintaining balanced electrolytes since your body will naturally become depleted of these minerals as you sweat. It is also the main reason that sports drinks are popular. These drinks contain all the electrolytes the human body requires, allowing people to refuel on both water and minerals simultaneously. However, if you consume too many sports drinks or electrolytes in other forms, you will overload your blood and kidneys. It is important to contain a balance of electrolytes with neither too few nor too many.

Your kidney provides other functions. Some of them are:

- electrolyte levels and blood pressure maintenance

- excess acid elimination

- hydration control

- hormones and vitamin D production.

When the kidneys aren't able to purify and filter blood, it accumulates waste in the body, which is harmful. This condition is referred to as renal failure, and it can even cause death unless treated on time. Before understanding what, renal failure is, you need to understand what kidneys are. The two bean-shaped organs located on either side of your spine in your back are referred to as kidneys. They help in cleansing the blood by removing waste products from it in the form of urine. Not only this, but kidneys also help in maintaining the balance of certain elements in blood like sodium, potassium, and calcium, and even control the secretion of hormones that help in controlling blood pressure and red blood cells.

Kidney or renal failure refers to a condition where the kidneys aren't functioning like they are supposed to. "Kidney failure" covers a lot of different problems, and some of these problems could be an insufficient supply of blood to your kidneys for filtration. Diseases like diabetes, high blood pressure, and any damage to the kidney's filters can+ severely damage your kidneys. Any scar tissue or even kidney stones can block your kidney and result in renal failure.

Some different signs and symptoms can help you spot kidney failure. It is important to be aware of these symptoms because early detection can help in timely treatment and curb the problem before it becomes severe. Keep an eye out for the following signs if there is a decrease in the output of urine over some time, retention of any fluid that results in the swelling up of your legs, ankles, or feet, extreme drowsiness, and shortness of breath, feeling of constant fatigue, confusion, seizures or even coma in some severe cases, a build-up of pressure in chest or chest pain. Also, there are cases where acute kidney failure causes no signs or symptoms and can be detected through different lab tests done for some other reason. You should immediately make an appointment with your doctor when you start noticing any of the signs or symptoms of acute kidney failure.

The Kidneys and the Endocrine System

The human kidneys play an important role in the endocrine system, which is the production and control of hormones within the body. The kidneys are critical in the production of the hormone renin, erythropoietin, and calcitriol. Not only that, but they also synthesize prostaglandins, which affect various aspects of kidney function.

Along with the production and synthesis of hormones, the kidneys also participate in the degradation of hormones, including insulin and the parathyroid hormone.

Erythropoietin:

The erythropoietin hormone regulates the production of red blood cells. When this hormone is out of balance, a person's blood can either become dangerously thin or dangerously thick, potentially lethal if left without emergency medical intervention.

For adults, an average of ninety percent of their erythropoietin is formed and synthesized by the kidneys. The liver produces the remaining ten percent. While the liver plays a vital role in erythropoietin production during the fetal stages of growth, for adults, the liver is no longer able to compensate for the kidneys' lack of production. That means that if the kidneys fail to produce adequate erythropoietin levels, the liver cannot maintain this hormone's healthy levels.

Most people who develop end-stage renal failure will experience anemia and a deficiency in erythropoietin. While doctors will sometimes administer blood thickeners to increase red blood cell production, it is not always effective.

Calcitriol:

Also known as 1,25-dihydroxy vitamin D3, calcitriol is a vital bioactive form of vitamin D3. This vitamin has important roles in bone mineralization and health, phosphorus regulation, and calcium regulation. However, many calcitriol effects are yet to be discovered, as they reside in various cells.

Calcitriol is important for human health, as the body cannot directly benefit from vitamin D absorbed from food or the sun. This "vitamin" is not a true vitamin but is instead a hormone. The vitamin D we absorbed from outside sources is delivered to the kidneys, synthesized into the bioactive form of calcitriol. Once the calcitriol has been synthesized, it can then be used by the body to maintain homeostasis.

As kidney disease frequently causes a deficiency in calcitriol, many doctors will treat their patients with this hormone. In can be used to treat symptoms such as:

- Hyperparathyroidism, an endocrine disorder characterized by excessive hormone production.
- Low blood calcium
- Osteomalacia, softening of the bone.
- Osteoporosis, degradation of the bones.

Calcitriol has a couple of other purposes, as well. First, it activates cell osteoblasts. This cell secretes the matrix needed for bone formation and synthesizes collagen required for nearly all tissues, cartilage, and many other body aspects. Second, calcitriol stimulates the small intestine, allowing it to synthesize protein then and absorb calcium.

Renin:

A part of the angiotensin-aldosterone system (RAAS), renin is an important component in kidney hormone health. After all, this system manages fluid balance, electrolyte balance, blood pressure, and systemic vascular resistance.

When there is a decrease in blood volume in the kidneys (causing low blood pressure) due to insufficient blood flow, your cells will begin to synthesis the renin protein and enzyme. The renin releases and alters several different enzymes and proteins, resulting in creating angiotensin II. That then causes the arteries to constrict, resulting in a rise of both diastolic and systolic blood pressure. Therefore, renin plays a vital role in raising low-blood pressure to a safe and manageable level.

Prostaglandins:

The cellular metabolism of arachidonic acid derives the prostaglandins from creating a series of fatty acid hormone-like products. Unlike most hormones, prostaglandins are not produced and then carried through the bloodstream to affect the body's specific functions. Instead, they are created by chemical reactions throughout the body wherever they are needed at the time. These prostaglandins' purpose is to help the body heal from both illness and injury, making them a part of the inflammation response.

While chronic high inflammation levels are damaging, as we will discuss later in this book, the inflammation response is still a vital part of the body. Without the inflammation response, we would be unable to heal or protect ourselves from harmful bacteria and viruses. They also manage blood clotting when we get a wound to be less likely to bleed out. Not only that, but prostaglandins play an important role in the female reproductive system. This hormone controls the menstrual cycle, ovulation, and induction of labor.

But if prostaglandins are produced throughout the body as needed, what do they have to do with the kidneys? The kidneys are one of the many locations within your body that produce this hormone, and it plays an important role in kidney health. It turns out that the prostaglandins produced within the kidneys play an important role in overall kidney function. The kidneys' process of filtering waste, delivering minerals to the bloodstream, adding clean fluids back to the bloodstream, and transporting urine to the bladder is known as renal hemodynamics. Pro prostaglandins help manage this entire process. Without renal prostaglandins, the kidneys would be unable to function properly, creating dangerous side effects.

As you can see, the kidneys play several very important roles in overall health. That means that it can be quite dangerous when something goes wrong with the kidneys, causing extreme symptoms. But what exactly could go wrong with your kidneys? First, when your kidneys are unable to function correctly, it can cause a build-up of fluid and waste within the body, along with excessive levels of minerals and electrolytes. This would result in kidney disease, which can, later on, lead to high blood pressure, fluid retention, fatigue, and back pain.

Many things may cause the kidneys to become damaged or diseased. Some of the causes may be infections, various diseases, diabetes, or high blood pressure. The kidneys can also become damaged if there is a malfunction of the blood vessels leading to the kidneys, causing the organs to receive inadequate blood supply. As there is no one cause of kidney disease or damage, your doctor will have to diagnose your kidney disease itself and the cause of the disease. Your doctor must learn the initial cause; otherwise, they will be unable to treat it properly. For instance, if your kidneys are damaged due to the inadequate blood supply, your doctor will be unable to help if they are only treating you for diabetes. Thankfully, your doctor should be well-equipped to learn the cause of your disease if you have one.

Chapter 2: Chronic Kidney Disease (CKD)

What is Chronic Kidney Disease (CKD)?

We talk about Chronic Kidney Disease (CKD) when kidney functions decline for three months or more. There are five stages of evolution of a CRM according to the severity of the renal involvement or the degree of deterioration of its function.

Sometimes failure suddenly occurs. In this case, it is called an 'acute failure' of the kidney, which is often treated with urgency by dialysis for some time. Usually, kidney function recovers itself. Generally, this disease settles slowly and silently, but it progresses over the years. People with CKD do not necessarily go from stage 1 to stage 5 of the disease. Stage 5 of the disease is known under the name of end-stage renal disease (ESRD) or kidney failure in the final stage.

It is important to know that the expressions terminal, final, and ultimate mean the end of any kidneys' function (kidneys working at less than 15% of their normal capacity) and not the end of your life. In order to stay alive at this stage of the disease, it is necessary to resort to dialysis or a kidney transplant. Dialysis and transplantation are known as renal replacement therapy (TRS).

That means that dialysis or the transplanted kidney will "supplement" or "replace" the sick kidneys and do their job.

What Are the Causes of Chronic Kidney Disease?

There are different kinds of diseases and disorders of the kidneys. At present, we do not know for sure all the causes. Some are hereditary, while others develop with age. They are often associated with another disease, such as diabetes, heart disease, or high blood pressure.

Most kidney diseases attack kidney filters, damaging their ability to eliminate waste and excess fluids. No treatment can cure these diseases, but it is possible to prevent them or slow down their evolution. It is especially true of diseases such as diabetes and hypertension, the leading causes of kidney failure.

The CKD is defined by the presence of an anatomical and urinary indicator of renal impairment and a decrease in the rate of glomerular filtration (GFR) persisting beyond three months. This disease is classified into five stages of increasing severity, according to the GFR. A DFG within normal limits characterizes the first two stages. It requires renal impairment markers, including urinary tests (proteinuria, Haematuria, or pyuria) or morphological abnormalities renal ultrasound (contours bumpy, asymmetrical in size, small kidneys or large kidneys, polycystic, etc.).

A real decrease in GFR characterizes only the other three stages. The end-stage of chronic renal failure (CRT) or stage 5 of the CKD is defined by a GFR <15 ml/min / 1.73 m^2.

Renal impairment is defined by the presence of pathological abnormalities or biological markers of the kidney, including abnormalities of urinary or kidney morphological tests detected by imaging.

Historically, the lack of consensus in the definition of CKD (especially chronic renal failure), its severity has led to late diagnosis, inadequate medical management, and data deficiency at a global level.

It was not until 2002 that this gap was filled by adopting the DFG thresholds or the CKD stages mentioned above.

Even though people with diabetes use insulin by injection or take medication, they cannot shelter some small blood vessel lesions, like those in the eye's retina. In this case, the retina may be damaged, resulting in loss of vision. Also, they are not immune to the deterioration of the fragile blood vessels of the renal filters.

Progressive deterioration of the kidneys is seen when urine tests show higher and higher protein levels. As the disease progresses, the number of protein increases. As for treatment, the sooner it starts (for example, with drugs such as ACE inhibitors or A2 blocking agents), the more likely it is to slow the disease's progression. Kidney disease caused by diabetes can slow the evolution of the disease regardless of its stage.

Over time, diabetes can reach kidney filters at a point of no return: the kidneys no longer function, and renal replacement therapy becomes essential. People with diabetes are prone to infections, which are changing rapidly. If these infections, especially those of the urinary tract, are not treated, they can damage the kidneys. It is recommended that people with diabetes not overlook any condition and have it treated immediately.

Hypertension

The kidneys secrete a hormone that plays an important role in increasing or reducing blood pressure. When the kidneys are so affected that they do not function properly, this hormone's secretion can increase and cause hypertension, damaging the kidneys. Therefore, it is necessary to closely monitor hypertension to avoid renal function deterioration in the long term.

Glomerulonephritis

The glomerulonephritis, or nephritis, declares when glomeruli, these little tiny filters used to purify the blood, deteriorates. There are several kinds of glomerulonephritis. Some are hereditary, while others occur as a result of certain diseases such as strep throat. The causes of most glomerulonephritis are not yet known. Some glomerulonephritis cure without medical treatment, while others require prescription drugs. Some do not respond to any treatment and who have chronic kidney disease. Some clues suggest that glomerulonephritis is due to a deficiency in the immune system of the body.

Autosomal Dominant Polycystic Disease

Often in their forties, people with the disease will need dialysis or a kidney transplant. But because the loss of kidney function is changing at a different pace, depending on the individual, the time between the onset of cysts and the need for dialysis varies widely. Since the disease is hereditary, people are advised to inform other family members to carry out the required tests as they may be affected.

The Obstruction of the Urinary Tract

Any obstruction (or blockage) of the urinary tract may damage the kidneys. Blocks can occur in the ureter or at the end of the bladder. Narrowing the ureter at the superior or inferior level is sometimes due to congenital malformations, leading to chronic kidney disease in children. In adults, increased prostate volume, kidney stones, or tumors often obstruct the urinary tract.

Reflux Nephropathy

The reflux nephropathy is the new name of the former "chronic pyelonephritis."

Illegal Drugs

The use of illegal drugs can cause kidney damage. Over-the-counter medications (without a prescription) High-dose and long-term use of over-the-counter medications can cause kidney damage.

Important: Beware of medications, including herbal remedies, sold without a prescription. It would be wiser to seek the advice of your doctor before buying them.

Prescription Drugs

Some medications prescribed to people with kidney disease cause renal dysfunction. The lesions are sometimes reversible and sometimes irreversible. Many medicines prescribed by prescription are safe but provided the doctor makes changes accurate to the dosage. So always ask your doctor or your pharmacist, information about potential side effects of prescribed drugs.

Other Kidney Disorders

Other issues can affect the kidneys, such as, for example, kidney stones, Syndrome Alport, Fabry disease, Wilms tumor (children only), not including infections of bacterial origin.

What are the complications of chronic kidney disease?

- Fluid in your lungs or fluid retention that might cause swelling in your legs and arms
- Blood vessel and heart disease
- High blood pressure
- Hyperkalemia
- Increased risk of bone fractures and weak bones
- Anemia
- Reduced fertility
- Erectile dysfunction
- Decreased sex drive

- Decreased immune response
- Central nervous system damage, causing seizures, personality changes, and difficulty concentrating
- Pericarditis
- Irreversible damage to your kidneys
- Pregnancy complications

Stages of Chronic Kidney Disease (CKD)

Chronic kidney disease (CKD) is not a sudden condition; it occurs in stages. Patients move from one stage of chronic kidney disease to the other as the kidneys' effectiveness decreases over time until they get to the last stage. The last stage of chronic kidney disease is kidney failure. At this stage, patients need dialysis or a kidney transplant to survive.

Stages of chronic kidney disease are identified according to a patient's estimated Glomerular Filtration Rate (GFR) - the rate at which the kidney filters toxins from the blood. GFR is considered the yardstick for measuring overall kidney functions. GFR is usually determined by examining the level of blood creatinine. This waste product is produced during muscle metabolism, in conjunction with other factors such as age, sex, body size, and race. . Let us highlight the stages of chronic kidney disease (CKD).

Stage 1

At stage one, the kidneys' functions are still normal, and patients may not notice any obvious symptoms. But protein can be noticed in patients' urine if tested. The estimated glomerular filtration rate (GFR) of the kidneys at stage one is 90 ml per minute or above. This is similar to the GFR of a healthy kidney.

Stage 2

Stage two chronic kidney disease (CKD) characterizes a mild decrease in kidney functions. At this point, a little rise in creatinine level in the blood can be noticed if the patient is tested. The estimated glomerular filtration rate (GFR) of the kidney in stage two is around 60 to 89 ml per minute.

Stage 3

Stage 3 is often referred to as the middle stage of chronic kidney disease (CKD). It is the most common category of chronic kidney disease. At stage 3, there is a moderate decrease in kidney functions, and patients must have started to sense some complications of chronic kidney disease. These complications include anemia, high blood pressure, bone weakness, and fatigue. The third stage of chronic kidney disease (CKD) occurs in two phases. The estimated glomerular filtration rate (GFR) for phase one, stage 3 of CKD is around 45 to 59 ml per minute, while phase two features an estimated GFR of 30 to 44 ml per minute.

Stage 4

At stage four, the kidney functions will have decreased immensely, and the patient will be faced with a lot of negative health conditions associated with chronic kidney disease (CKD). This stage is associated with severity. At this stage, doctors will already be planning for dialysis or a kidney transplant. The estimated glomerular filtration rate (GFR) in stage four is around 15 to 29 ml per minute.

Stage 5

Stage five is the last stage of chronic kidney disease. It is the stage where the kidneys finally fail. The estimated glomerular filtration rate (GFR) is below 15 ml per minute. The kidneys may still be able to function a bit, but the kidney function level at this stage will not be enough to keep the patient alive. At stage five, the patient will need dialysis or a kidney transplant to survive.

Chapter 3: Kidney Failure

What is kidney failure?

You reach the "Kidney Failure" stage when your kidneys cannot remove toxins and waste in your blood from the foods you eat and the things you drink. Sometimes called "chronic kidney disease" or "chronic kidney failure."

It isn't a disorder that happens overnight— it's a gradual issue that can be discovered early and treated, diet modified, and it's possible to solve what causes the problem.

Partial renal failure is possible, but it typically takes a long time (or really bad diet for a short time) to achieve full renal failure. You don't want total renal failure because it will require regular dialysis to save your life.

Specifically, dialysis procedures wash excess blood and pollutants in the blood using a device because your body can no longer do the job. Despite therapies, death could be very painful. Renal failure can result from long-term diabetes, high blood pressure, an irresponsible diet, and other health concerns.

A renal diet is about moderating the diet's protein and phosphorus intake. Limiting sodium intake is also necessary. By regulating these two factors, you can regulate most of your body's toxins/waste, improving your kidney function.

When you notice it early enough and control your diet with extreme care, you can avoid complete renal failure. When you notice it early, you can remove it.

It's your kidney's job to remove stuff you don't need and balance the ones your body needs. If your kidneys couldn't play this role effectively, it's high time you discover what you can do. A doctor's prescribed renal diet can help filter out toxic substances you don't need in your body.

Understanding the Different Types of Kidney Failure

In general, there are five different kidney failures that you should be aware of. I will try to go through them one by one to clear things up.

1. Acute Pre-Renal Kidney Failure

It is caused by insufficient blood flow to the kidney. In this scenario, the kidney fails to filter the blood toxins as enough blood doesn't flow through it. It is possible to treat this type of failure as long your doctor can figure out the cause of your abnormal blood flow.

2. Acute Intrinsic Kidney Failure

It can happen if you experience any form of direct trauma to your kidneys, such as an accident or physical impact, causing toxins to overload and might lead to ischemia (Oxygen fails to get enough oxygen).

Some causes include:

- Shock
- Bleeding
- Glomerulonephritis
- Renal Blood Vessel Obstruction

3. Chronic Pre-Renal Kidney Failure

It happens when your kidney fails to receive sufficient blood for a prolonged period. In this situation, the kidney tends to shrink, eventually losing its function.

4. Chronic Intrinsic Kidney Failure

It occurs if your kidney has experienced long-term damage due to intrinsic kidney disease.

Intrinsic diseases can come from a lack of oxygen, bleeding, or trauma.

5. Chronic Post-Renal Kidney Failure

If you experience blockage in your urinary tract for a long time, then the pressure build-up might damage your kidney.

Understanding if Your Kidneys Have Failed

There are various ways to understand if your kidneys have any problems.

Some of the common ones include:

- *Urinalysis* → In this type of test, the doctor will take samples of your urine and check them for any abnormalities, such as sugar or abnormal protein that might have leaked into the urine.

- *Urine Volume Measurements* → Measuring your urine volume is possibly one of the simplest tests out there. If you have very low urine output, it might indicate that you have kidney disease caused by a urinary blockage.

- *Blood Samples* → If urine isn't doing it, the doctor might ask you to take blood tests to measure various substances filtered by the kidneys.

- *Imaging* → Various imaging tests, such as CT Scans, MRIs, and Ultrasounds, tend to provide a full image of the kidney and the urinary tract, allowing the doctor to find blockages or abnormalities.

- *Kidney Tissue Samples* → Tissue from your kidney can be taken and examined to look for scarring, toxin deposits, or infectious organism. The physician will try to take a kidney biopsy to collect your sample.

In most cases, the doctor will take a biopsy sample while you are awake; however, the doctor will give you a local anesthetic to ensure that you don't feel any pain.

Acute Renal Failure - Symptoms and Treatment

Acute renal failure (ARF) is a very serious but treatable condition resulting from kidney function loss. There are various symptoms and treatments for acute renal failure or otherwise known as acute kidney failure.

Acute kidney failure, as stated earlier, is sudden kidney function loss. As you may know, your kidneys are responsible for removing body waste products and helping balance other minerals in your body and bloodstream.

They're an essential part of the body, as the body can't work without them. If your kidneys stop working in acute kidney failure, the body will quickly fill up with many waste products, contaminants, and other liquids, rendering it lethal.

How is Acute Renal Failure Caused?

Acute renal failure has various causes. Many are related to other factors in the body that can affect the kidneys, while others are directly related.

Urine-flow Blockage.

It can cause kidney failure by blocking kidney waste excretion. It can be caused by a tumor, enlarged prostate, blockage or inflammation of the urinary tract, trauma, or kidney stones.

Blood loss to the kidneys.

Any type of body injury, but more specifically localized kidney injury, can cause sudden blood flow loss, resulting in severe kidney damage.

Some medicines can cause acute kidney failure.

Some medicines can have some very large side effects on the kidneys. Many of these medicines can be found in some antibiotics, blood pressure medicines, certain colors used in CT scans, and more commonly, some pain killers.

All these can have a poisoning effect on the kidneys and should not be taken for extended periods. When you suffer from any of these problems, try to find other ways to cope, including finding ways to fix the problem's first cause.

Some people may risk more acute kidney failure. Those suffering from chronic conditions such as heart conditions, obesity, liver disease, high blood pressure, and other organ conditions will have more acute renal failure.

Also, as mentioned earlier, it is important to explore ways of reducing pressure on the kidneys when suffering from the above condition to avoid any chances of acute renal failure or kidney disease.

What are Acute Renal Failure's common symptoms?

Before any type of kidney disease is apparent, signs can be seen and considered very mild, and some may even remain unnoticed until too late. If you have any of these common symptoms, act immediately.

Common symptoms of acute renal failure may include:

- Fluid retention (swelling in the body—usually feet and hands)
- Loss of appetite
- Urinating problems
- Some vomiting and nausea
- Dizziness
- Lower back pain
- And general restlessness.

In people already suffering from other long-term medical conditions, these signs may go unnoticed and may be thought to be related to the current disease. It is important to remember that steps should be taken to help treat the condition at the slightest sign of acute renal failure symptoms.

Simple medical tests decide how to tell if you have acute kidney failure. After consulting the doctor, urine and blood samples must be taken.

These can help show your blood and urine toxicity and help you decide if you are now at risk of acute renal failure. Other measures, such as measuring the fluid intake and loss, are very important to determine whether fluid retention is caused.

Acute renal failure has some forms of treatment, including hospital stays and continuing procedures. All this depends on the severity of acute renal failure and signs and causes of renal problems.

Such therapies vary from dialysis, medicines, and surgery. Based on how far the renal failure can go, appropriate medication is selected.

Nevertheless, most physicians now believe that acute renal failure is largely caused by poor diet and lifestyle factors, as with virtually all medical conditions. Some of our preferred Western foods contain preservatives and chemicals that our bodies cannot process.

They usually contain large amounts of sodium and potassium, which are not good for anyone fighting kidney disease. The kidney diet was created based on eastern diets (which now have very rare genetic-related renal failure) and has been shown to help treat and even reverse acute kidney failure.

Learning to Deal with Kidney Failure

Learning that you are suffering from kidney failure might be a difficult thing to cope with. No matter how long you have been preparing for the inevitable, this is something that will come as a shock to you.

It might be a little bit difficult at first to get yourself oriented to a new routine, but once you get into the groove, you'll start feeling much better.

Your nurses, loved ones, doctors, and co-workers will all be there to support you.

To make things easier, though, let me break down the individual types of problems you might face and how you can deal with them.

Chapter 4: Causes of CKD

Causes and Risk Factors

Many of us are not aware that the cause of kidney disease doesn't necessarily have to occur in the kidneys themselves. Problems affecting our overall health and well-being can also induce damage to the kidneys. In the same way, common health problems can also impair the function of these organs. The most frequent causes of kidney disease are hypertension and diabetes.

High blood pressure, which affects 75 million people in the US or one in three adults, can damage blood vessels in the kidney and impair their function. In other words, damage to blood vessels in the kidneys due to hypertension doesn't allow them to remove wastes and extra fluid from your body. That leads to a vicious cycle as an accumulation of waste, and extra fluid increases blood pressure. Besides damaging filtering units in kidneys, high blood pressure can also reduce blood flow to these organs. As you're already aware, without a blood supply, organs cannot function properly.

About 30.3 million people, or 9.4% of the United States population, have diabetes, causing several complications. Just like hypertension, diabetes also damages small blood vessels in the kidneys. As a result, the body retains more salt and water than it should. Moreover, diabetes also damages the body's nerves, making it difficult for you to empty the bladder. The pressure from a full bladder can back up and damage or injure kidneys. Let's also not forget that if urine remains in the body for a long time, it can lead to an infection from the fast growth of bacteria and high blood sugar levels. Estimates show that 30% of patients with type 1 diabetes and 10% to 40% of people with type 2 diabetes will eventually experience kidney failure.

Besides diabetes and hypertension, other causes of kidney disease include:

- Infection
- Renal artery stenosis
- Heavy metal poisoning
- Lupus
- Some drugs
- Prolonged obstruction of the urinary tract from conditions such as kidney stones, enlarged prostate, some cancers

Diagnosing Kidney Disease

Your doctor will be the first to know if you are in a high-risk group for getting kidney disease. They will do some tests to see how well your kidneys are functioning. Some of the tests might be:

Urine Test

Your doctor will ask for a urine sample to test it for albumin, a protein that gets passed into the urine if the kidneys become damaged.

Kidney Biopsy

When doing a kidney biopsy, your doctor will take out a little piece of tissue from the kidney after being sedated. This sample could help determine if you have kidney disease, what type you have, and the amount of damage that has already happened.

CT Scan or Ultrasound

A CT or computed tomography scan and ultrasound can give your doctor clear pictures of your urinary tract and kidneys, letting your doctor see if your kidneys are too large or small. They can also show any structural problems or tumors that might be there.

GFR or Glomerular Filtration Rate

This test measures how well the kidneys work and shows what stage of kidney disease you might be in.

Chapter 5: Symptoms of CKD

One way to help a person know if he or she is suffering from chronic kidney disease is to be informed about its signs and symptoms.

When these signs and symptoms show, immediately seek the assistance of medical experts to avoid complications.

The common signs of chronic kidney disease are:

- **Nausea and Vomiting.** When you experience nausea, you sense discomfort in your upper stomach. You get a sensation of uneasiness and an urge to vomit involuntarily. Most of the time, a person vomits after experiencing nausea.

- **Loss of Appetite.** Changes in your eating habits may be a sign that you are already suffering from chronic kidney disorder. When you begin to notice that you are eating less than usual or are not feeling any urge or motivation to eat at all for no apparent reason, it is time that you consult your doctor. Not only is it a sign of chronic kidney disease, but loss of appetite may also result in weight loss and malnutrition.

- **Changes in urination.** Whether you are urinating more or less than usual or are experiencing changes in your urine's color, you should seek medical assistance. We know for a fact that the kidneys are the ones responsible for the production of urine. If there are changes in urination, this means that there are changes in the functioning of the kidney as well. It may be a sign of improvement for some but can be very risky for many. You know that you are experiencing changes in urination when you frequently need to wake up in the middle of the night just to urinate, your urine has a bubble or is foamy, when it contains blood, dark-colored. You urinate less frequently and in smaller amounts, or whenever you feel difficulty or pressure when urinating.

- **Swelling.** Swelling may occur whenever you are injured or when you accidentally bumped into something hard. However, if you experience swelling without any external cause, then this may be a sign that your kidneys are beginning to fail. Swelling occurs because the kidneys are no longer able to remove the extra fluids in your body. Swelling may occur in the ankles, legs, feet, hands, or face.

- **Fatigue**. The kidneys produce hormones responsible for keeping us energetic every day. When they fail, our bodies also fail to receive and carry oxygen, making our brains and muscles tire quickly.

- **Itching or Skin Rash**. As mentioned in the first chapter, one of the kidneys' main functions is to filter the blood and remove the bloodstream wastes when the kidneys fail to function properly; these wastes build-up, causing itching and skin rash.

- **Shortness of Breath**. When the kidneys fail to remove extra fluid in our body, they can stay in the lungs and build up in there. Kidney can also trigger the development of anemia. When anemia is complicated, your body will starve for oxygen. Thus, one experiences shortness of breath.

- **Trouble concentrating and dizziness**. As mentioned earlier, different parts of the body fail to receive and carry oxygen due to kidney failure. One of these is the brain. If the brain fails to get enough oxygen, you may experience dizziness, memory problems, and inability to focus properly.

Other minor signs may be:

- Weight loss

- Blood in urine

- Insomnia

- Muscle cramps

- Erectile dysfunction in men

Now that you know the signs and symptoms of chronic kidney disease, it is easier for you to detect whether you are suffering from it or not. However, knowing the signs and symptoms is not enough.

Chapter 6: Correlation With Other Diseases

According to experts, the renal disease requires early diagnosis and targeted treatment to prevent or delay both a condition of acute or chronic renal failure and the appearance of cardiovascular complications to which it is often associated.

Hypertension and diabetes, not adequately controlled by drug therapy, prostatic hypertrophy, kidney stones, or bulky tumors, can promote onset. They reduce the normal flow of urine and increase the kidneys' pressure and limit functionality.

Or the kidney damage can be determined by inflammatory processes (pyelonephritis, glomerulonephritis) or by the formation of cysts inside the kidneys (polycystic kidney disease) or by the chronic use of some drugs, alcohol, and drugs consumed in excess.

A fundamental role in alleviating the already compromised kidneys' work is the diet, the first prevention. It must be studied with an expert nutritionist or a nephrologist to maintain or reach an ideal weight on the one hand and on the other to reduce the intake of sodium (salt), and the consequent control of blood pressure, and other substances (minerals), without creating malnutrition or nutritional deficiencies. Particular attention should also be paid to cholesterol, triglycerides, and blood sugar levels.

Understanding what causes kidney failure goes a long way to deciding just what kind of treatment you should focus on. The most important factor that you should focus on is, of course, your diet. But as you focus on your diet, make sure that you are following your doctor's instructions in the event of other complications. Let us look at a few of the common causes of kidney diseases.

Diabetes

Time for a crash course in diabetes.

Diabetes causes damages to the different organs in our bodies, including:

- Heart
- Kidneys

- Eyes
- Blood vessels
- Nerves

What many may already know is that diabetes affects our body's insulin production rate. But what many may not know is the extent of damage that diabetes can cause to the kidneys. Insulin is essential because it regulates the level of sugar or glucose in our blood. The inability to control the glucose damages the kidneys' function to filter fluids and waste products.

We do know that diabetes is one of the leading causes of CKD. But we have yet to understand in detail why and how it can harm the kidneys.

High Blood Pressure

When blood pressure increases and has become uncontrollable, it causes stroke, heart attack, and chronic kidney disease. Too much pressure against the blood vessels' walls can contribute to the kidney's failure to function properly.

Thus, a person must watch over his diet and the activities he engages in to avoid hypertension. Although it is a common health problem, it still poses serious risks and complications.

The risk factors for hypertension include age, obesity, family history, smoking, lack of exercise, stress, excessive alcohol consumption, high fat diet, and sodium intake.

An important thing to remember here is that high blood pressure can be both a cause and CKD symptom, similar to diabetes.

So, what exactly is blood pressure? People often throw the term around, but they cannot pinpoint what happens when the blood pressure increases.

Autoimmune Diseases

IgA nephropathy and lupus are two examples of autoimmune diseases that can lead to kidney diseases. But just what exactly are autoimmune diseases?

They are conditions where your immune system perceives your body as a threat and begins to attack it.

We all know that the immune system is like the defense force of our body. It is responsible for guiding our body's soldiers, known as white blood cells, or WBCs. The immune system is responsible for fighting against foreign materials, such as viruses and bacteria. When the system senses these foreign bodies, various fighter cells, including the WBCs, are deployed to combat the threat.

Typically, your immune system is a self-learning system. That means that it can understand the threat and memorize its features, behaviors, and attack patterns. It is an important capability of the immune system since it allows the system to differentiate between our cells and foreign cells. But when you have an autoimmune disease, your immune system suddenly considers certain parts of your body, such as your skin or joints, as foreign. It then proceeds to create antibodies that begin to attack these parts.

Before one thinks about his or her condition treated, it is first important to know the causes and symptoms. Knowing the causes of a particular disease is necessary in treatment and prevention.

Chronic kidney disease is most commonly caused by hypertension and diabetes. 2/3 of the cases of chronic kidney disease are found in people suffering from these two conditions. However, other factors may account for the development of chronic kidney disease.

Malformations

Even when you are still in your mother's womb, risks of developing chronic kidney disease are already present. Mothers should be extra cautious when pregnant because preventing urine outflow may affect the baby's organs.

Lupus

Systemic lupus erythematous causes the body's immune system to attack the kidney even if it is not a foreign tissue. It may take a long time before a person recovers from lupus because it eventually goes back after some time, but it is possible through proper treatments.

Obstructions

Obstructions or blockages such as tumors, kidney stones, or enlarged prostate gland can trigger chronic kidney disease development.

The causes mentioned above are just the most common of the many causes of chronic kidney disease. There are cases when CKD is caused not only by a single factor. Sometimes, a combination of these factors causes the development of chronic kidney disease.

Nonetheless, a patient needs to know the cause of their condition to be prescribed with the proper treatments and medications.

Kidneys may be small, but they do have important functions in the body. These bean-shaped organs work hard, but they may experience injuries and other problems that prevent them from functioning properly. But the question is, what causes kidney disease and how to detect it?

Chapter 7: Conventional Treatments

Dialysis

It is an artificial way of filtering the blood that gets used when your kidneys are very close to failing or have completely failed. Most people who have kidney disease might have to go on dialysis totally or until you find a kidney donor. Dialysis is a treatment that is performed to filter and purify the blood using a specialized machine. A dialysis machine performs the same function as the human kidneys. Depending on your condition's severity, you may be required to undergo dialysis treatment once a week or 2-3 times weekly. People should understand that dialysis treatment doesn't cure the disease; it only helps you extend your life.

There are two kinds of dialysis: **peritoneal** and **hemodialysis**.

Peritoneal Dialysis

In this type of dialysis, the peritoneum starts functioning for the kidneys. The peritoneum is the membrane that outlines the abdominal wall. A tube gets implanted and is used to fill the stomach with dialysate. All the waste in the blood will flow out of the peritoneum and into this dialysate. This fluid then gets drained out of the stomach.

There are two types of peritoneal dialysis:

1. **Continuous cycler-assisted peritoneal dialysis:** for this one, a machine is used to pull the fluid in and out of the stomach while you sleep.

2. **Continuous ambulatory peritoneal dialysis:** for this one, the stomach is filled and then drained numerous times throughout the day.

The common side effects are infection of the stomach cavity or around the area where the tube was inserted. The other side effects could include hernias and weight gain. A hernia happened when a part of the intestine pushed through a tear or weak spot in the stomach wall.

Hemodialysis

Hemodialysis is a type of dialysis that is performed with the use of a dialysis machine. Blood will be passed into the machine via a tube connected to an "access" (we shall talk about "access" later under this subtopic). The machine will then filter the blood to eliminate excess fluid and waste products from the blood. There is a part of the dialysis machine called the dialyzer. The dialyzer acts as a filter during hemodialysis. It is modeled after the glomeruli. The dialyzer ensures that toxins and waste products are filtered out of the blood while protein and red blood cells, which are too big to escape the filter, are retained. After filtration, clean blood containing protein and red blood cells will be released into the blood via another tube. Patients usually undergo hemodialysis thrice a week. Each hemodialysis session can last up to four hours or more, depending on the amount of waste in the blood and the dialysis machine's capacity. Hemodialysis is the most preferred dialysis treatment for most kidney failure patients.

Kidney Transplant

A kidney transplant is another option that can be used to treat kidney failure. A person who received a new kidney can go back to their normal routine, and dialysis is no longer needed. It is normally a long process before a person with kidney failure can get a compatible donor. After the transplant, you are required to take immunosuppressive drugs to prevent your body from rejecting the newly introduced kidney. A kidney transplant may not be for everyone, especially for those who have compromised immunity. It is best to talk to your doctor about this procedure.

One amazing thing is that our body can function well with just one kidney. When a person's kidneys fail, another person can donate one of their healthy kidneys to the kidney failure patient. After the kidney transplant, the patient and the donor can live a healthy life with one healthy kidney. In some cases, the donor may be deceased; healthy kidneys can be removed from someone who just died to replace a kidney failure patient. Thus, we have two categories of kidney transplantation: living-donor kidney transplantation and deceased donor kidney transplantation. Living donors are usually close relatives of the patient. To receive a healthy kidney from a deceased donor, you have to be on a national waiting list. The procedures for benefiting from deceased donor transplantation may vary across countries.

Drugs and medication

Your doctor will either endorse angiotensin-converting enzyme (ACE) inhibitors, for instance, ramipril and lisinopril, or angiotensin receptor blockers (ARBs, for instance, olmesartan and irbesartan). However, medicines for blood pressure can slow the movement of kidney disease. Your doctor may recommend these medicines to save kidney work, regardless of whether you have hypertension.

You may likewise be cured with cholesterol drugs (for instance, simvastatin). These remedies can reduce blood cholesterol levels and assist kidney health. Relying upon your side effects, your doctor may also recommend medications to relieve expansion and treat anemia (decline in the number of red blood cells).

Medical Management

Suppose you have budget issues or j want to avoid dialysis or transplant altogether. In that case, there are some medical solutions that you might look into to reduce the symptoms of kidney failure.

They won't completely reverse the effects, but they might let you stay healthy until your kidneys can no longer function.

If you opt for medical management, then the first thing to do is consult with your physician, as they will point you in the right direction.

They will create a care plan to guide you on what you should do and what you should not do. Make sure always to keep a copy of the plan wherever you go and discuss the terms with your loved ones as well.

It should be noted that most individuals who tend to go for medical management opt for hospice care.

The primary aim of hospice care is to decrease your pain and improve your final days' quality before you die.

In medical management, you can expect a hospice to:

- Help you by providing you with a nursing home

- Help your family and friends to support you

- Try to improve the quality of your life as much as possible

- Try to provide medications and care to help you manage your symptoms

- But keep in mind that regardless of which path you take, always discuss everything with your doctor.

Chapter 8: Dr. Sebi and Kidney's Health

How did dr. Sebi address kidney diseases?

Dr. Sebi said, "Detoxification is at the heart of getting rid of kidney problems associated with mucus out of the body; there are no other ways that will bring the required result." Therefore, fasting is an essential factor that can help detoxify the body, especially the kidney. Fasting helps your body, including the blood, kidney, and liver, to experience cleansing and detoxification. To achieve a cure for kidney problems, you have to be willing to make a sacrifice like the one you are about to undergo.

Detoxifying your body could end your kidney problems, depending on how serious you engage in the methods, since they are not easy to eliminate.

Some of Dr. Sebi's products used for cleansing and detoxification are Bio-Ferro, Viento, and Chelation. You can buy them in drsebiscellfood.com.

Any problem with your kidneys might lead to your blood not being purified well. It causes toxins to be accumulated in the blood. You might have a family history of kidney problems, high blood pressure, and diabetes. Recent studies show that overusing normal medications for various diseases can significantly deteriorate your kidneys' health. Many people are habitual users of medications, even for the slightest aches and pains. You have probably done it since you didn't know that these drugs could harm your health, including your heart, liver, and kidneys. Many people today have moved to a more holistic approach to their health. Dr. Sebi knew what some scientists are trying to prove today. He might have known that people today would need his help in curing their kidney problems. Yes, he created an herbal remedy for kidney problems.

If you have been diagnosed with kidney disease, following Dr. Sebi's diet can help you. Make sure you talk with your doctor if you feel like something isn't quite right with your health. When you think about all the toxins being put into our bodies today, it isn't any wonder that there are so many people with kidney problems.

Treatment and Passing of Kidney Stones

The treatment of kidney stones requires the intake of alkaline herbs beneficial for consumption as food and medicinal herbs. That means you have to consider both methods to be able to fight kidney abnormalities and problems.

The diet, which comprises vegetables, fruits, and grains, contains high amounts of magnesium and calcium because a reduced amount of these minerals could result in kidney stones problems.

Herbs can are very effective for fighting stones, and some of them are also very common

The herbs perform their functions by relieving edema in the ureter mucosa, decreasing spasms that occur due to kidney stones' irritation, and improving urine flow.

Examples of these herbs are:

1. **Saw Palmetto Fruit**

Saw palmetto fruit contains many ethyl esters of fatty acids, enzymes, tannins, resins, terpenoids, and sitosterols.

It is a reliable plant used for the treatment of Benign Prostate Hyperplasia (BPH). The herb contains a tonic that helps the urinary tract, and it is used for both male and female sufferers.

This fruit contains spasmolytic effects, making it easy to remove stones, and it also benefits patients with dysuria and tenesmus. This herb reduces the bladder's pressure and has a sedative effect on an irritated detrusor, which assists sufferers with bladder and prostate abnormalities.

2. **Dandelion Leaf**

This plant leaf is very effective in the detoxification of the liver and kidney. The leaf is a strong diuretic, and it is compared to furosemide in animal studies. It has also been carried out in humans, and it was discovered that the effects are similar. Animal studies have shown that dandelion leaf is important in removing kidney stones via the direct passage.

Dandelion is one of the major sources of potassium, with about 4.25% potassium compared to other drugs, containing a lesser amount. It can be used as a diet and medication because of its ability to improve its urinary and biliary system.

3. **Lobelia Flower, Seed, and Leaf**

Lobelia contains powerful relaxant and antispasmodic effects that assist the urinary stones to pass through the ureters easily. This plant is regarded as acetylcholine antagonists though other mechanisms may speak for its broncho and ureter-relaxing effects.

4. **Goldenrod Leaf or Flower**

This herb is used as a strong urinary stimulant, improving diuresis and reducing albuminuria in the kidney.

It is also very important for nephritis treatment and helps stabilize the body immediately after the kidney has discharged the stones. That means it should be used immediately after the kidney stone has been ejected.

The presence of flavonoids in the plant helps repair the kidney, blood vessels, and connective tissues surrounding the kidney.

5. **Horsetail Leaf**

Horsetail leaf effectively repairs connective tissues surrounding the kidney and the lungs due to a silica component.

Horsetail also helps in diuresis, and it is a general metabolic stimulant that increases connective tissue resistance. It is important in both acute and chronic removal of kidney stones.

6. **Khella Seed**

Khella plant, especially the seed, contains khellin and visnadin as their active components, making it useful by acting as a mild calcium channel blocker in the ureters' dilation.

Visnadin contains some smooth-muscle relaxing components which is associated with the non-standard calcium-channel activity.

The active components present in Khella seed are excellently absorbed and have reduced toxicity as evidenced by the almost total lack of side effects with long-term use in treating an individual with asthma.

7. **Corn Silk**

Corn silk is a very important herb as it is used to increase the easy flow of urine. It contains a demulcent property that helps reduce irritation from stones and facilitate its easy removal.

This plant should be collected fresh, especially when it is still very green, to prevent the consumption of a low-quality herb.

8. **Madder Root**

Madder root is significant and used by patients with kidney problems because it has a spasmolytic effect on the ureters and enables the free passage of stones. This plant was studied, and it has been proved to contain calcium-channel antagonizing effects, which might contribute to relaxing the muscles.

This plant is also used to prevent calcium and phosphate oxalate salts from forming kidney stones in the body.

9. **Gravel Root**

This plant is used for the treatment of the urinary tract.

Gravel root can dissolve concretions. It is used for the treatment of urethritis, cystitis, irritable bladder, and fluid retention.

10. Horse Chestnut Fruit

This plant is used to treat various health conditions because of anti-edema properties known as escin. Escin reduces the small pore number and diameter in capillary endothelium, thereby decreasing fluid seepage into the tissues (Longiave D. et al. 1978).

The presence of calculi in the ureter is easily removed with the use of this plant. The plant has anti-edema properties that help in the production of enlargement of the internal diameter of the ureter, thereby helping the stones to migrate easily even in resistant cases.

11. Couch Grass

This plant is a saponin and mannitol-containing diuretic that contain some silica. This herb helps in the repair of irritated mucous walls and has been used to treat prostatic adenoma.

This plant helps in the easy removal of stones and helps repair and prevent kidney stones' recurrence.

12. Hydrangea Root

This plant is important and useful for the easy removal of stones. It is also helpful for sufferers who have urinary tract infections and prostate enlargement.

Foods to Limit to Safeguard Kidney Function

We have already seen a lot of the food that you should avoid. For that reason, I am going to include a few more to the list, explain why they should be avoided, and then I am going to show you some incredible spice blends and seasonings that you can use on your food. And to make things even more interesting, I will show you some lip-smacking sauces and kitchen staples that are perfect for the renal diet.

Let's start with some foods that you should avoid.

Whole-Wheat Bread

Normally, whole-wheat bread is considered a healthy option. But for people with kidney diseases, that is not the case. The reason for this is that the more whole-wheat and bran in bread, the more potassium and phosphorus content you are likely to find in them.

A 30 gram (or 1 ounce) serving of whole-wheat bread could contain around 68 mg of potassium and 57 mg of phosphorus, and if you eat plenty of it, that would potentially be too much for your kidneys.

Brown Rice

The case for avoiding brown rice is similar to the one made to avoid whole-wheat bread; it contains too much potassium and phosphorus for your body to handle. A single cup of brown rice contains about 154 mg of potassium and around 150 mg of phosphorus. Compare that to a cup of white rice, and the difference is remarkable; you will find just 54 mg of potassium and around 68 mg of phosphorus in the white rice. That's less than half the amount that brown rice has!

If you feel that you do not want to include white rice into the diet, try alternatives to brown rice such as couscous, bulgur, buckwheat, and pearled barley. They are not only nutritious but delicious as well.

Dairy

Milk is often recommended for strong bones and muscles. But for those with kidney diseases, having milk increases the potassium and phosphorus content in the blood. It might be important for people to consume milk in many cases since it aids them with other medical conditions. If you require milk in your diet, ensure that you communicate your medical history, issues, current diet, and other vital information to your doctor. By doing so, you will get proper recommendations on how you can include milk in your diet.

When you visit your doctor, make sure that you are completely honest about your medical history, habits, and diet. Don't try to hide the fact that you occasionally sneak in a cup of that good, sweet, chilled soda pop in the middle of the night. Don't be embarrassed to admit something if it concerns your kidneys or your health. Your doctors are not there to judge you. Trust me; there is nothing you can say that they haven't seen or heard before. And in some cases, what they might have experienced could be quite shocking or surprising to you.

Alkaline foods you should include in your daily diet

Alkaline foods help counter the potential risks of acidity and acidity refluxes, bringing some kind of relief. The majority of traditional Indian foods contain alkaline foods to make a balanced diet.

If you have indulged in excessive reddish meats and processed foods, isn't it about time you included some alkaline food in what you eat? Here is a list to truly get you started.

Green Leafy Vegetables

The majority of green leafy vegetables are thought to come with an alkaline effect inside our system. It isn't without reason our elders and wellness experts always recommend us to add greens to our daily food diet. They contain important minerals that are essential for your body to handle various processes.

Cauliflower and Broccoli

They contain several phytochemicals that are crucial for the body. Toss it up with various other vegetables like capsicum, coffee beans, and green peas, and you possess your health dosage right there.

Citrus Fruits

Contrary to the fact that citric fruits are highly acidic and could have an acidic influence on your body, they will be the best way to obtain alkaline foods. Lemon, lime, and oranges contain Vitamin C, and so they are recognized to assist in detoxifying the machine, including providing rest from acidity.

Seaweed and Ocean Salt

Did you know seaweed or ocean vegetables have 10-12 times more mineral content material than those grown on land? They are also regarded as highly alkaline meal sources and so are known to produce various advantages to the body program. You can suggest adding nori or kelp to the plate of soup or make sushi at home. Or simply sprinkle some ocean salt into the salads, soups, omelets, etc.

Root Vegetables

Underlying vegetables like fairly sweet potato, beets, and carrots are excellent resources of alkali. They taste greatest when roasted with just a little sprinkling of spices and additional seasonings. Frequently, these are overcooked, making them miss out on almost all their goodness. Consider while cooking, and you'll fall deeply in love with root vegetables as you figure out how to use them in soups, stir-fries, salads, and more.

Seasonal Fruits

Every nutritionist and wellness expert will let you know that adding seasonal fruits to your diet can benefit your well-being. They come filled with nutritional vitamins, nutrients, and antioxidants that look after various stomach functions. They may be good alkaline meal sources too.

Nuts

Don't you love to chew on nut products when food cravings activate? Besides being resources of great fats, also, they create an alkaline impact in the stomach. However, being that they are high in calorie consumption, it's important to have limited nut products. Add cashews, chestnuts, and almonds to your daily meal strategy.

Onion, Garlic clove, and Ginger

Being among the most important ingredients in Indian cooking food, onion, garlic, and ginger are excellent flavor enhancers. You should use them in different ways – garlic clove to liven up your early morning toast, grated ginger within your soup or tea, newly sliced up onions in salads, etc....

Chapter 9: Avoiding Dialysis

Many people are habitual users of medications, even for the slightest aches and pains. You have probably done it since you didn't know that these drugs could harm your health, including your heart, liver, and kidneys. Many people today have moved to a more holistic approach to their health. Dr. Sebi knew what some scientists are trying to prove today. He might have known that people today would need his help in curing their kidney problems. Yes, he created a herbal remedy for kidney problems.

If you have been diagnosed with kidney disease, following Dr. Sebi's diet can help you. Make sure you talk with your doctor if you feel like something isn't quite right with your health. When you think about all the toxins being put into our bodies today, it isn't any wonder that there are so many people with kidney problems.

Ingredients in the Kidney Disease Kit

Dr. Sebi's kit combines many very healthy and rare herbs that he thought was perfect for any kidney problem. Unfortunately, not all problems can be treated with the same herbs. Dr. Sebi's kits let you customize them for your needs. Let's look at the ingredients:

- **UTI Special Mix**: UTIs are the most common problem with kidneys. If you are constantly getting UTIs, this might help you stop getting them.

- **Kidney Stone Hunter**: This herbal mix works against kidney stones. Even if you don't get kidney stones, this can help detoxify your body.

- **AHP Zinc Powder**: AHP or ayurvedically herb purified zinc powder can be taken by anyone with a zinc deficiency. Zinc deficiency can cause kidney problems.

- **Swarna Bang Tablets**: This combination of herbs has been used for thousands of years to fight recurring UTIs. These are strong enough to help the kidneys, too.

- **Punarnava Special Kidney Mix**: Some reports published about kidney disease claims punarnava is one herb that helps the kidneys function properly.

As you know, your kidneys are a critical filtration part of your body. Without it, we wouldn't survive for long with all the toxins we are exposed to every day. Even with the slightest of imbalances in filtering out toxins, we could face cysts, kidney stones, UTIs, gout, or other chronic and severe complications. Some are fairly common, but others can be life-threatening.

Dr. Sebi's kidney kit gives your body the minerals and herbs your body needs to keep your kidneys healthy. They can help your body function better by detoxifying your body. The herbs help to cleanse the kidneys of all the toxins it has stored up. That won't happen overnight; it will take several months for you to notice any results. Each kit will last for about two months.

When you go to Dr. Sebi's website, there will be some questionnaires for you to feel out. These will help them pick the right combination of herbs for you. You will then get to decide what you want to try to improve your health.

Chapter 10: Dr. Sebi Method to Heal Kidneys

Dr. Sebi's Official method for treating Chronic Kidney Disease, such as any other disease, is composed of 3 main steps. Please note that any of these parts can't be passed over to succeed in your healing journey.

The three steps I'm talking about are:

1. **Cleansing** → The body must be cleansed on an intra-cellular level through detoxification to purify each cell and remove the excess of mucus.

2. **Revitalizing** → After cleansing, you need to nourish your body to regenerate your cells and strengthen the immune system.

3. **Keeping the Body Healthy** → Follow Dr. Sebi's nutrition guide and adopt healthy lifestyle habits every day to keep your mind and body in good shape.

1. Cleansing

How to Prepare Cleansing Herbs?

Preparing your cleansing herbs would depend a lot on the form you purchased them. It's easier to prepare cleansing herbs that come in powder forms, as you can easily make herbal teas with them in the specified or recommended dosage. However, for other forms form herbs, especially roots or leaves, it is better to use a ratio of 1 teaspoon to 1 cup (8 oz) of spring water for each herb.

However, for easier batch preparation and storage, I recommend preparing herbs in batches of mixtures. That would mean mixing them up according to function and benefit. Again, this will depend on the state of your health and what minerals are most important for you. You can combine similar herbs with similar functions into a batch. Like our healer, Dr. Sebi would say: *"If you want calcium, you know where to go to (sea moss), if you want Iron, you go to Burdock, and if you want a mix of both Iron and Fluorine, you go to Lily of the Valley"*.

In all, try not to mix more than 2 or 3 herbs. Remember, these herbs are electric, and it's best to preserve their organic carbon, hydrogen, and oxygen nature as much as we can. Again, if you mix more than that, you may not get their accurate concentrations per ml of water, so try to limit it to 3, possibly 2.

For a clearer understanding, you can use the following mix:

- Mix **Colon and gallbladder** cleansing herbs together

- Mix **liver and kidney** cleansing herbs

- Mix **respiratory and mucus cleansing** herbs

- Mix **lymphatic and heavy-metal** cleansing herbs.

Since these herbs perform a whole-body cleanse (not just colon), including the skin, eyes, colon, liver, lymphatic system, and gallbladder, you can decide to choose how to combine them. Also, note that when you make larger batches of these herbs for storage, try not to make batches that last more than 7 to 14 days.

For pre-purchase cleansing packages
Please follow the recommended dosage or instructions that are provided for that cleansing package

For fresh Green leafy herbs
- Place in spring water and boil on low heat for 5 to 7 min

- For dried leafy herbs, boil longer – 10 to 15 min

For Dried ground (or powder) herbs
For dried ground or powder leaves or roots, mix in recommended ratios for the herb. Powder herbs are the easiest to mix in dosage proportions, so you can simply follow the package instructions

For Chunks of Dried Root herbs
If you've purchased chunks of roots or stems, you can prepare them in the following way:

- Cut or break up chunks

- Place in spring water and boil for 15 minutes

- Let cool and serve

- Alternatively, prepare in larger batches and place in jars to store in the refrigerator.

For bulk purchase herbs

If you have purchased herbs in bulk and you're making your teas, find out what the recommended dosage is for each herb. As a general rule, you should prepare each herbal tea ratio of 1 teaspoon to 8 ounces of spring water.

For capsules

I recommend that you do research and find out what the recommended dosage is for each herbal capsule

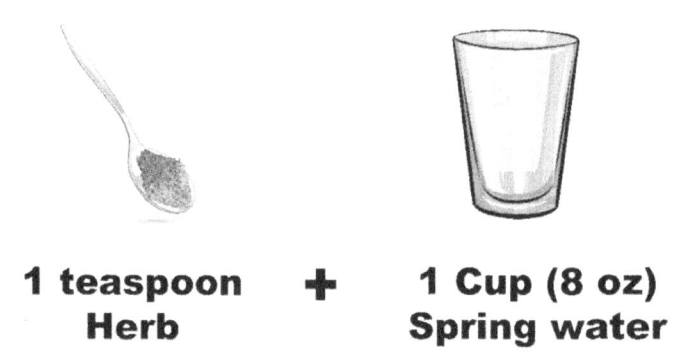

1 teaspoon Herb + 1 Cup (8 oz) Spring water

How To Take The Prepared Cleansing Herbs

If you are on medication, I recommend taking the herbs one hour before taking your meds; Dr. Sebi recommended this. Your colon cleansing herbs should not be consumed for longer than 30 days because your body may become dependent on them, and you want to start to reduce the dose during your last 3 to 5 days, depending on how long you've been taking them.

Routine:

- **Twice a day** - morning and night

- **Daily Consistency** - Try to stay consistent both in terms of timing and duration. That is, try not to skew the duration. Make it consistent, and take the cleansing herb throughout the cleanse. For example, for a 14-day cleanse, the cleansing herbs can be taken twice daily, and you should take them around the same time you do take them on both mornings and evenings.

- **Gradual Wean Off** – Just like medications, it is not the best to go cold-turkey when it comes to herbal detox. Towards the end of the cleanse duration, wean off your herbs by gradually reducing the dosage and duration. The duration of the wean will depend on the length of the fast you choose. For example, for a one month fast, I usually start weaning a week towards closure. For a 14 day fast, I begin weaning on day 11 or 12. You can begin the wean by reducing it from twice a day to once a day. Or simply take half the dosages each for mornings and night.

You must do this because you need to signal to your body to begin to prepare to start functioning independently without dependence on the cleansing herbs. And no other way to do this than to take it slow and gradual, without bringing too much "shock" to your body.

How to break a detox fast?

- Slowly reintroduce solids

If you are doing water or a liquid fast, you will need to reintroduce solid foods slowly. You can begin by introducing solids like high water-content fruits. These include watermelon, apples, and berries. After that, you can proceed to introduce softer fruit solids like bananas and avocados. Later, you can incorporate more harder solids like veggies. All foods must be listed on the nutrition guide. However, if doing a fruit or raw veggie fast, you can break the fast right away on solid foods.

- Drink 1-gallon spring water daily

Drink spring water daily together with the revitalizing herbs and sea moss.

How long should you detox/cleanse?

How long you should detox depends on your state of health, that is, your body's toxification level (the less healthy you are, the more toxic your body is) and tolerance level. Typically, it is recommended to fast for 7-14 days, but Dr. Sebi recommends a minimum of at least a 12 day fast. Dr. Sebi himself fasted for 90 days to cure himself of diabetes, asthma, and impotence. It is great to cleanse at least once a year for 7 days if you consume an alkaline diet. If you are not consuming an alkaline diet, then you should cleanse/detox every 3 months

I fasted for 14 days, and I would recommend fasting for between 14 days and 1 month if you have high blood pressure. Again, your body's tolerance level will ultimately determine the length so, watch your body and study its reaction as you begin the fast. We are all different, and you may find that you cannot handle a basic liquid fast (water or juice). In that case, you can get started with fruit or raw vegetables fast. But make sure all foods and fruits are listed in the Dr. Sebi Nutrition Guide. Whether liquid, juice, or raw food fast, the results are virtually all the same – the only major difference is when it takes to begin to see results. While raw food fasts take longer, liquid fasts are much faster. So do not worry; the most important thing is to stay committed and focused on whatever fasting method you choose.

Common Symptoms Expected During Detox Cleanse

- Cold and Flu symptoms
- Changes in Bowel movements
- Fatigue and Low Energy
- Difficulty sleeping
- Itching
- Headaches
- Muscle aches and pains
- Acne. Rashes and breakouts
- Mucus expel (catarrh, etc.)
- Lower blood pressure

If you relate to any of these symptoms during the cleansing stage, be happy. That's because your body is pushing out all the toxins and mucus you have been keeping inside for so long. These symptoms are only temporary and usually resolve after the first one to two weeks.

Herbs to Take During Detox

Prodigiosa

Prodigiosa, also known as 'Prodijiosa or Hamula, is a perennial plant with large bushy leaves and flowers, and it's from the daisy family and native to Mexico and California. These plants have a grey-purple hue on the underside and dark green leaves on the upper side and grow up to 5 feet in height with its flowers growing in clusters. This plant has a long history with the Mexicans as it has been used for centuries to treat diabetes, arthritis, diarrhea, and stomach disorder and relieve aching joints.

Because of the chemical and compound composition of Prodigiosa, research has it that it is very effective for the treatment of diabetes II because of how it aids in stimulating the pancreatic gland to secret and reduces or lowers blood sugar level and burn down fat in the gallbladder. The irony is that Prodigiosa can cause more damage to people that are suffering from Type I diabetes. Furthermore, consuming Prodigiosa's tea/infusion helps boost the digestion of fat and improve the synthesis of bile in the liver, dissolve tiny gallstones, and treat chronic gastritis and other digestive systems disorders. Although there is no research to prove its effectiveness in treating cataracts, it is believed that it can cure cataracts.

Prodigiosa is used for several reasons, included:

- Treatment of diabetes (type II).
- Treatment of diarrhea.
- Treatment of stomach pain.
- Treatment of gallbladder disease.
- Enhancing the digestion of fat and boosting the digestive system's healthiness.

The note-full precautions to beware of before using or consuming Prodigiosa includes:

- Pregnant and breastfeeding mothers should not use or consume Prodigiosa as there is no research to back it if it is safe or not.
- It is a no-go area for people suffering from diabetes I., and people with diabetes II should control their sugar level while consuming this herb.

How to prepare Prodigiosa tea/infusion:

1) Dry the fresh leaves until it is dried.
2) Once the fresh leaves are dried, or the one you ordered for is available, boil 8 or 16ounce of water and brew 1 or 2 tablespoons of Prodigiosa leaves in the warm water for 15minutes.
3) After brewing it, strain the Prodigiosa leaves.

4) Take a cup (8ounce) of Prodigiosa tea/infusion two times per day for the dosage.

Burdock Root

Burdock root is the root of a delicious plant called Burdock, which all its body or parts are useful as either food or medicine. This plant can be found all over the world. I called this plant the wonder plant because everything about it is important as we consume its root as food, and we also use it for medicinal purposes, and both its leaf and seed are used for medicinal purposes.

For over five centuries, people worldwide have been using burdock root orally to treat and prevent various health disorders.

Because of Burdock root's chemical composition, such as; quercetin and luteolin, research has it that it can serve as a great effective antioxidants that can treat and prevent cancer by preventing cancerous cells from growing and mutating and also combat aging. Compound like 'Phytosterols' helps boost scalp and hair follicles to grow healthy hair even from baldhead. The vitamins-C helps in boosting the immune system and combat bacterial. It also helps to cleanse or detoxify the liver and lymphatic system, etc.

The potassium helps reduce blood sugar levels and filter the blood by removing impurities through the bloodstream and eradicating toxins through the skin and urine.

The benefits of using or consuming burdock root tea/infusion include:

- cleanse/detox the liver and lymphatic system.

- treat and prevent diabetes by reducing blood sugar levels in the body.

- eliminate toxins from the body by inducing sweetness and urine.

- purify the blood by removing heavy metals from the bloodstream.

- treat various skin disorders and combat aging.

- treat and prevent cancer by inhibiting the growth and mutation of cancerous cells.

- boost the immune system and enhance circulation.

Till at the time of writing this book, there are no side effects that have been recorded by researchers or people that have used these herbs.

However, research has it that applying this root to your skin might cause rashes.

For the dosage and how to prepare Burdock root tea/infusion, kindly take the following steps:

1) Scrub the uprooted root of burdock heartily under running water to remove all the dirt that accompanied it from the soil.

2) You should chop the Burdock root into smaller pieces (less than 1 inch). Please note that if you order it online, it will come dried and already chopped.

3) Pour 2-3 cup of water into your saucepan and add ¼ cup of the chopped burdock root and boil it.

4) Once the water is boiling, lower your gas, re-boil it for 30-40 minutes, and put off your gas.

5) Once it is cold, strain it and consume it.

6) For the dosage, drink one glass cup daily

Bladderwrack

Bladderwrack is a type of brown algae or seaweed typically found in the chilly waters of the Northern Atlantic and Pacific coasts of the United States and on the Atlantic and Baltic coasts of Europe.

Although bladderwrack has been growing in cold ocean waters for thousands of years, its use as a health-supportive supplement is relatively recent.

Some of the known benefits of this algae are the following:

- Promotes healthy mineral levels

- Supports a healthy hormone balance
- Supports a healthy metabolism and a healthy weight
- Seeks to support the immune system
- Boost the energy levels

Dosage and administration:

Bladderwrack may be eaten whole or made into a tea using 1 teaspoon per cup of hot water, allowing each cup to sit at least 10 minutes before drinking. You can drink up to three cups of tea per day.

Dandelion

Dandelion is a flowering plant known as 'yellow gowan' or 'lion's tooth'. This plant is native to Eurasia and today. It is common in over 60 countries worldwide in the mild climates of the northern hemisphere. For centuries, these flowering plants have been used for the treatment of swelling (inflammation) of the pancreas, relieve pains that are caused by inflammation, treat and prevent cancer, tonsils (tonsillitis), skin disorder, bladder or urethra disorder, digestive and liver problems and enhance the general health of the liver and digestive system.

Researchers proved that it is a very effective cleansing/detoxification herbs because of the chemical compositions and nutrients.

The benefits of using or consuming Dandelion include:

- It helps to detoxify or cleanse the liver and the kidney.
- It helps to treat and prevent diabetes by regulating blood sugar levels.
- It helps to fight against and relieve pains that are caused by inflammation.
- It helps to deactivate and inhibit the negative effects of free radicals in the body, which is because of its antioxidant properties.

- It reduces the level of cholesterol.

- It lowers blood pressure by getting rid of excess fluid in the body.

- It helps to naturally shed excess weight gain by improving the metabolism of carbohydrates.

- It helps in boosting the digestive system.

- It helps to boost the immune system.

- It helps to keep the skin healthy and treat and prevent skin diseases.

Till at the time of writing this book, Dandelion is 100% safe, but consuming an overdose of it can result in some side effects like:

- Experiencing stomach upset or irritation

- Allergic reactions

The special precautions before using/consuming dandelions are:

- Pregnant and breastfeeding mothers should stay off dandelion as there is no research to know if it is harmful to them or not.

- If you are suffering from Eczema, stays off dandelion as more than 85% of people with eczema suffer an allergic reaction to dandelion.

For the dosage and how to prepare Dandelion tea/infusion, kindly take the following steps:

1) Get some fresh leaves of dandelion and washed it under running water to remove all the dirt.

2) After washing it, pour ½ - 1 cup of the washed dandelion into your saucepan.

3) You should boil 4-5 cups of water and pour the boiled water inside the saucepan where you pour the dandelion and cover it for 12-15 hours or throughout the night (overnight).

4) The next day, strain out the dandelion leaves, and you will be left with the dandelion tea/infusion.

5) For the dosage, take ½ tablespoon of Dandelion per ¾ cup of water three times daily. And if you ordered your dandelion online, you can take 4-10 grams of dry leaf of dandelion three times daily.

Elderberry

Elderberry is a dark purple berry from the elder tree, also known as European Black Elderberry or Sambucus Bacchae. This plant is a flowering plant from the family of Adoxaceae and native to Europe. Both the leaves and fruit (berries) of elderberry have been used for centuries to treat pain and swelling arising from inflammation. It also helps to stimulate urine production and induce sweat to detoxify the body system.

Because of how rich elderberry is with various compounds and nutrients like vitamin-C, dietary fiber, phenolic acids, which is a great and powerful antioxidant that helps to prevent and decrease the damage that is caused by oxidative stress in the body, it also contains some compound like flavonols such as kaempferol, quercetin, isorhamnetin and anthocyanins which gives the fruit the black-purple color and makes it a strong antioxidant and anti-inflammation agent.

Elderberry also contains some nutrients, like:

- Calories
- Carbs
- Minute amounts of protein and fat
- And anthocyanins, making the plant a strong and effective antioxidant with anti-inflammatory properties.

The benefits of using/consuming elderberry include:

- It helps cleanse and detoxify the lungs and respiratory system by eliminating mucus from the upper respiratory system and the lungs.
- It helps to treat constipation.
- It helps to treat flu and cold in less than 24hours.

- It combats harmful bacteria in the body by preventing bacterial growth through its antibacterial properties.

- It boosts and supports the immune defense system by increasing white blood cell production.

- It protects and keeps the skin healthy.

- It helps to relieve chronic fatigue syndrome and depression.

Till at the time of writing this book, there is no record of any side effects from researchers and people who have used elderberry, but because of the compound that are presents in elderberry, it will be wise to use it for not more than 12 weeks and take a break for at least a week before using it again.

The notable precautions before using elderberry include:

- Ensure children below 12 years do not use/consume elderberries, and children above 12 and less than 18 should not use it for more than 10days.

- Since there is no reliable information to know if elderberries are safe or not for pregnant and breastfeeding mothers, I strongly advise that they stay off elderberries.

- People who have a history of suffering from an autoimmune disease like; multiple sclerosis, lupus, rheumatoid arthritis, etc., should stay off elderberry as it has the potency to boost the immune system become more active, which could worsen their situation.

- Since elderberries have the potency to increase or boost the immune defense system, any medications designed to decrease the immune system's function will certainly interact with Elderberry.

For the dosage and how to prepare Elderberry tea/infusion, kindly take the steps below:

1) Boil 8-12oz of water in your saucepan.

2) Once the water is boiling, measure one tablespoon of dried elderberries and add it to the boiling water.

3) Reduce your gas and allow it to boil for at least 15 minutes.

4) After the 15 minutes timing, allow it to get cold and strain it using a strainer.

5) For the dosage, consume 3-4 cups daily.

Sarsaparilla Root

Sarsaparilla root is the root of a tropical wood climbing vine that belongs to the genus Smilax family. Dr. Sebi recommends it as a revitalizing herb for many diseases, including cancer, because it is very rich in iron, calcium, and phosphate.

The benefits of consuming Sarsaparilla roots are:

- It helps to destroy and prevent cancerous cells from mutating.

- It binds the endotoxins responsible for the lesions in psoriasis patients and eliminates them from the body system.

- It helps to fast-track healing and recovery.

- It treats and prevents health issues that are caused by inflammations like: joint pain, swelling of any parts of the body, arthritis, rheumatoid, etc.

- It soothes and heals sexually transmitted diseases such as syphilis, herpes, gonorrhea etc.

- It helps to treat and prevent leprosy

- It helps to protect and reverse damages done to the liver to function perfectly.

- It makes the body absorb nutrients and other herbs easily

When writing this book, there are no side effects attributed to this herb's consumption. However, because of the 'saponins' that it contains, I advise you to consult your doctor before using this herb as saponins can cause stomach irritation.

For the dosage and how to prepare sarsaparilla root tea, kindly take the following steps:

- Harvest some sarsaparilla plant roots and wash it under running water to remove all the dirt that accompanied it from the soil.

- After washing it, pill off the outer skin, chop it into smaller pieces, and dry it in a well-ventilated place (indoors) for at least seven days (ensure you turn the drying root daily for the seven days until it is completely dried.) iii. Once it is dried, store it in a paper bag or cardboard box. (Ensure you don't store it in a plastic container as it will get mold).

- Measure 1teaspoon of the dried chopped Sarsaparilla root and add it to your saucepan and add 8 ounces of water. Boil it for 15-20minutes v. Strain it using a strainer. You are done!

- For the dosage, consume 1cup (8ounce) 3 times daily.

Guaco

Guaco is a climbing plant with different names like Huaco, Guace, or Vejuco. This climbing plant belongs to Asteraceae and cordifolia species' family and is very rich in numerous minerals and compounds. Its leaves are very medicinal and nutritional that the people of Aztecs use them for cleansing the blood system and clearing heavy metals from the bloodstream.

There are a lot of benefits that one can benefit from using or consuming Guaco. Some of them are:

- It lessens the effect or symptoms of snake poison.

- It is used to thin the blood through the coumarin activities it contains (anticoagulant and blood-thinning.)

- It helps to combat inflammation through its anti-inflammatory properties.

- It treats stomach irritation through the effect of its cleansing activities.

- It helps to treat respiratory disorders like coughs, rheumatism, bronchitis, etc.

- It enhances quick recovery from the wound.

- It helps to cleanse or detoxify the blood and skin by clearing heavy metal from the blood.

- It boosts and builds the immune defense system.

- It can treat some infections diseases such as; candida yeast infection, herpes, etc.

Until writing this book, there are no severe side effects that researchers or uses have recorded.

Like I said earlier, Guaco is 100% safe for consumption by mouth, but if you are taking or using any Coumadin drugs, please consult with your doctor before using it.

And if you have any history of bleeding, do not use Guaco unless your doctor approves of it. Like I said earlier, Guaco helps to thin the blood, so any medications that can thin blood or slow blood clotting do interact with Guaco.

For the dosage and how to prepare Guaco tea/infusion, kindly take the following steps:

1) Get some handful of fresh Guaco and wash it under running water or 2 ounces of it dried leaves if you have the dried ones.

2) Pour about 6cups of water in your saucepan together with the Guaco leaves boil it until it is reduced to 2 cups.

3) You can add some brown sugar (optional) if you add the brown sugar; allow it to boil for another 20 minutes.

4) Strain the syrup with a strainer.

5) You should bottle it and store it in a refrigerator.

6) For dosage, take 1 soupspoon 3-4 times daily.

Eucalyptus Tree

Eucalyptus tree is a fast-growing evergreen tree that is a native of Australia. This plant's leaves and bark are used for various medicinal purposes like joint and muscle pain, cold, cough, congestion, etc. However, the Chinese, Greek, and Indian Ayurvedic people have incorporated this amazing herb to treat various types of conditions for thousands of years before now.

This plant/tree has more than 400 different species. The most used is the Eucalyptus globulus or the Australian fever tree, also known as Blue Gum.

Eucalyptus leaves cineole that is also known as eucalyptol, in which the leaf's gland contains an essential oil (eucalyptus oil) and also; flavonoids and tannins, which are plant-based antioxidants that aids in reducing inflammation, control blood sugar, fight against the activities of bacteria and fungi and the oil can help in relieving pain and inflammation as well as blocking chemicals that usually cause asthma.

The benefits of using or consuming eucalyptus tea/infusion include:

- Cleansing the skin through steaming/sauna.

- Relieving common cold symptoms like cough lozenges and inhalants and also sore throat and sinusitis

- Relieving symptoms of bronchitis. Inhaling the vapor of eucalyptus tea helps serves as a decongestant by loosening phlegm and easing congestion.

- It aids in relieving asthma: research showed that eucalyptus has the potency to break up mucous in people who have asthma.

- It aids in dental plaque and improves gingivitis

- It helps in improving bad breath

Until writing this book, eucalyptus leaves are 100% safe for consumption.

However, eucalyptus oil is not as safe as the leaves as applying the oil directly to the skin without diluting can lead to serious nervous system problems.

The precaution to be note-full of before using eucalyptus tea or infusion are:

- It is 100% safe for pregnant and breastfeeding mothers to consume eucalyptus tea or infusion

- If you are allergic to it oil, you might want to take some caution in consuming the tea as it might react to you.

- Before or after surgery, avoid consuming the eucalyptus tree's tea for two weeks as your blood sugar level might not be controlled.

- Since the eucalyptus leaf has the potency to lower blood sugar, consuming any diabetes medication can interact with eucalyptus tea/infusion.

For the dosage and how to prepare eucalyptus tea/infusion, kindly take the following steps:

- Boil water to 194-205 Fahrenheit. Alternatively, you can boil the water and drop it down for a minute or two to reduce the temperature.

- Pour a teaspoon of dried eucalyptus leaf into a teacup/mug.

- Pour 6 ounces of water inside the teacup/mug and allow the leaves to be steep for 10-15minutes.

- Get a filter to strain the loose leaves of the eucalyptus.

- You are a god. You can now enjoy the cup of eucalyptus tea/infusion at a go.

- For the dosage, take 3-4 cups per day.

Revitalizing

Revitalization is restoring, rejuvenating, and recovering all the energy that the body has lost due to the disease it has suffered from and during the cleansing period. According to Dr. Sebi, all the revitalizing herbs are rich in phosphate, calcium, iron, etc. The body needs a speedy recovery.

The recommended revitalizing herbs for kidneys health include:

Irish Sea Moss

Irish Sea Moss is red algae that belong to the family of Florideophytes that grows on the rocky parts of the Atlantic coast of various countries, including the British Isles, Jamaica, Scotland, etc. Dr. Sebi recommends this herb for revitalizing the body after cleansing because it has over 92 out of 102 minerals that the body needs to be healthy. Some minerals are, for example:

- Phosphorus
- Iodine
- Selenium
- Calcium
- Bromine
- Iron
- Potassium

Some of the benefits of consuming Irish Sea Moss are:

- It heal and boost the immune defense system.
- It treats and prevents hyperthyroidism and boosts the functionalities and health of the thyroid.
- It helps to soothe joint pain and swelling of the joint and treat arthritis.
- It helps to enrich the overall mood and reduce fussiness.
- It helps to combat infections caused by viruses and bacterial.
- It helps treat and prevent various skin disorders like acne, skin wrinkling, and alleviating inflammation.
- It helps to treat and prevent digestive and respiratory tract disorders.

The note-full precautions to beware of before consuming Irish Sea moss include:

- Because of how rich Irish Sea moss is with iron, it can trigger hypothyroidism for people suffering from Hashimoto's disease.
- Stop using the herb if you notice any allergies or reactions.

For the dosage and how to prepare Irish Sea Moss tea, kindly take the steps below:

- Measure and boil 1cups (8ounce) of water in a ceramic pot.

- Once the water is boiled, measure 2-3 tablespoon of Irish Sea moss gel (or 1teaspoon for the powdery form) and add it to the boiling water.

- Allow the Irish Sea moss for 10-15 minutes to dissolve completely.

You are done!

For the dosage, take 1cup of Irish Sea moss tea daily in the morning.

Contribo

Contribo is a unique herb. It grows along streams and in other wet areas. Even since it is notable for its use in western herbal medicine, we often find Contribo in Ayurvedic medicine and Traditional Chinese Medicine.

Various cultures around the world use Contribo for treating numerous diseases. Even ancient Greeks, Romans, and Byzantines have used it in their pharmaceutical recipes to treat various health conditions.

Their experts utilized this herb to treat conditions like:

- Kidney ailments
- Bladder stones
- Gout
- Snakebite
- Uterine complaints
- And insomnia

According to researchers, Contribo holds a lot more power than you can imagine. For example, when you infuse it in water and consume it, it gives your body immense power to fight cold and flu. Its properties are a lot more powerful and effective than many famous medicines.

Also, if you have some appetite issues, Contribo can assist in that as well. It enhances the appetite and aids in improving your overall health.

Dosage and Administration:

As a decoction: The usual daily dose is 3.10 g herb for internal use.
As a powder: 1-2 g daily for internal use.

Cordoncillo Negro

The cordincillo negro is a shrub whose leaves give off a spicy smell when squeezed and a bitter taste when chewed.

As a medicinal plant, the cordoncillo negro has several important uses. Before the plant can be used for medicinal purposes, its leaves are traditionally prepared in infusions and capsules.

Below are some of the curative uses of cordoncillo negro:

- **Cordoncillo can be used as a painkiller.** Chewing on the leaves of cordoncillo anesthetizes the mouth. So if you squeeze and rub these leaves over a cut or wound, it can serve as an anesthetic.

- **It can treat digestion problems** like vomiting, nausea, stomach ache, dyspepsia, dysentery, etc.

- **It can also prevent blood loss** from internal bleeding (uterine, gastric, pulmonary).

- **Cordoncillo can cure respiratory problems** like colds, flu, coughs, bronchitis, and pneumonia.

- **Helps to keep the kidney healthy** and prevent kidney stones

Dosage and administration:

Infusion: 1 cup 2-3 times daily (single dose: 1 g herb per cup; or 10% infusion: taken 3 or 4 times daily)

Hierba del Sapo

This herb has been traditionally used for centuries in Mexico and Central America to help treat kidney diseases and clear toxins from the arteries.

Some of the main benefits of this herb are:

- Antioxidant and anti-inflammatory properties

- Can help to lower cholesterol and triglyceride levels in the bloodstream

- Helps with gallstones and kidney stones

- Helps increase urine production to aid with kidney pain and swelling

Pao Pereira

Pao Pereira is a tree that belongs to the Apocynaceae family and native to South America. This tree's bark is very rich with various compounds that are very effective in destroying, eliminating, and inhibiting cancerous cells. Because of and how effective the bark of this tree is, Dr. Sebi recommends this herb to revitalize the body system after cleansing.

The benefits of consuming Pao Pereira include:

- treating malaria and other infections caused by parasites.

- It helps treat and prevent cancer by destroying cancer and preventing cancerous cells from mutation.

- Soothing and relieving liver pain.

- It helps to treat and prevent stomach disorders like constipation and irritation.

- It helps to boost sexual arousal

Till at the time of writing this book, there is no any side effect that is attributed to the consumption of Pao Pereira; but since there is no vital information to show that this herb is 100% safe for pregnant and breastfeeding mothers, I advise that they avoid this herb's consumption.

For the dosage and how to prepare Pao Pereira tea, kindly take the steps below:

- Harvest some Pao Pereira by cutting some of its bark without cutting down the tree, chopped it, and dried it.

- Once it is dried, boil 1liter of water and pour two tablespoons of the dried Pao Pereira into the boiling water.

- Lower the heat of the fire to a medium-low and place the lid on the pot.

- Boil the mixture under medium temperature for 20 minutes.

- Allow it to get cold and train it using a strainer or filter.

You are done!

For the dosage, consume 1 cup of the tea times daily.

Soursop

Soursop is the fruit of the "Annona Muricata" tree that is a native of tropical regions in the Americas that belongs to the Annonaceae family. Its leaves are widely used because they are rich with various nutrients like iron, calcium, phosphorus, magnesium, sodium, potassium, zinc, etc. That makes the tea very effective in fighting against the mutation of cancerous cells.

Other benefits of consuming soursops tea are:

- It helps to destroy and eliminate cancerous cells and inhibit the growth of cancer cells.

- It is a very strong and effective antioxidant that helps neutralize free radicals that can damage the cells.

- It helps to soothe heart disorders.

- It helps to lower blood sugar levels for people who have type 2 diabetes.

- It helps to fight against infectious diseases caused by bacterial. Such diseases like: yeast infections, cholera, gingivitis, Staphylococcus, tooth decay etc.

- It helps to soothe and alleviates swelling (inflammation) etc.

The note-full precautions before consuming of soursops tea include:

- Since there is no information about this herb's harmful effects on pregnant and breastfeeding mothers, I advise that they stay off this herb.

- Although this herb is tempting, please make sure you consume this herb under a medical practitioner's supervision.

For the dosage and how to prepare soursops tea, kindly take the following steps:

- Harvest some fresh Soursops leaves, dry it until it is dried, chop it, or pound it into smaller pieces. On the other hand, you can place an order online, and it will come dried and chopped.

- Measure 1 teaspoon of the chopped leaves of the Soursops and pour it into your teacup or mug.

- Boil 8 ounces of water and add it to the Soursop leaves in the teacup or mug and cover it.

- Allow the leaves to steep for 10-15 minutes and strain it.

You are done!

For the dosage, consume 2-3 cups of the Soursops tea daily.

Shepherd's Purse

Growing all over the world, it's one of the most common wildflowers on Earth. Its name comes from its small triangular fruits that resemble a purse, but it's also known as "lady's purse" or "mother's heart".

Among the conditions shepherd's purse is said to heal are:

- High blood pressure
- Bladder's infections
- Premenstrual syndrome
- Heavy periods
- Kidney diseases

Shepherd's Purse is certainly a safe herb to use for all ages; however, there are some doubts about its safety to use in pregnancy, and so it is best avoided at this time.

Dosage and administration:

The British Herbal Pharmacopoeia (BHP) suggests a dose of 1-4 gms or by infusion or a dose of 1-4mls of the ethanolic extract (a well-rounded tsp is approx 1.5 grams)

Herbal tea healing

Now you can begin your routine of herbal healing, which means you know how to use the food you consume as medicine to treat the things that ail you, the chronic conditions that lead to chronic diseases, and keep you in overall poor health. Herbal medicine is also known as herbalism, and it is based on consuming parts of plants to heal you.

Drinking teas made from herbs is one of the best and easiest ways to use herbs and plants for health, besides eating good food. You can also use plants in other ways for your health. You can infuse a part of a plant by steeping it in hot water for some time. When you add chopped bits of plants to cold water and allow it to stand and steep for longer periods, this is known as maceration. When using this method, the water will absorb the minerals from the plant parts. When you boil the roots or the bark of the plant, you have made a decoction. These methods can be used with any plant, and the liquid that comes from these methods will be full of minerals and vitamins that will keep you healthy.

You may already be using herbal preparations in your everyday life without knowing you are doing it. An extract is a preparation of herbs where tinctures are distilled into an extract. A tincture is made when you mix the herb with one hundred percent pure ethanol and allow it to be steep. The longer it steeps, the stronger the tincture will be. Completed tinctures have an alcohol content that will measure at least twenty-five percent. The percentage of alcohol in an extract is even less than the alcohol content of a tincture. So if you have ever cooked a dish that calls for pure vanilla extract, pure lemon extract, pure maple extract, etc., you have used an herbal preparation.

And while Americans are becoming better at using herbal medicines daily, the Asians and Europeans have centuries of practice to draw on. These are the things that Dr. Sebi tried to teach his followers. The art of being healthy goes beyond just eating healthy foods, although that is an important part of the equation. Everything you do for yourself must help to keep you healthy. People from China and India are particularly good at compounding herbs. This process refers to mixing several herbs in a particularly balanced formula to treat a specific problem. These are formulas that have been used for thousands of years and are quite effective in treating ailments. But the goal of using these compounds is not just to treat a specific disease or relieve a specific symptom. Botanical medicine aims to create changes in your body designed to make your body chemistry work better and better balance. A permanent cure and a healthier life can be achieved and maintained. And the particular compound used is generally tailored to that individual's particular needs, so no one formula is prescribed to all.

You will find many benefits to using herbal medicines besides the medicines themselves. Herbs will rarely have harmful side effects when used in the proper dosage, while many prescription medicines have adverse side effects that are often worse than those they are trying to treat. Medicines made from herbs will use the natural healing process of your own body to treat chronic conditions. The herbs you will be using are simple ingredients that are already made by your body. And herbal medicine is quite inexpensive, whereas modern medicine can be very expensive. Herbs are generally available almost anywhere. Some of the simpler herbs can be grown at home as people do in less industrialized parts of the world. You might not always know when you have already used a topical form of herbal medicine, but if you have ever used a lotion with aloe vera gel as one of the ingredients, you have used an herbal remedy.

Things that you use every day might have medicinal properties:

- **Ginseng** is taken as a tea to relieve respiratory and digestive issues.

- **Anise seed** is made into a tea to relieve chest congestion.

- **Basil** eaten with food will help settle a digestive upset and improve a sluggish appetite.

- **Black pepper** will stimulate your taste buds, stimulate your digestive systems so it will perform more efficiently, and clear out congestions of the lungs and sinuses.

- **Cayenne pepper** will stimulate your basic metabolic rate and help reduce bad cholesterol in your blood.

- **Chamomile** is gentle enough to use daily. As a tea, it will help you sleep, and when added to your bath, it will help you relax, and it will also help to soothe tired muscles.

- **Cinnamon** will help relieve heartburn and bloating, and it might help reduce your blood sugar levels.

- **Coconut oil** helps to increase your energy levels and to balance your hormones.

- **Cranberry** makes a delicious tea that will help prevent tooth decay and relieve your urinary tract problems.

- **Echinacea tea** will help prevent or treat infections of your throat or mouth and help relieve the symptoms of colds and sinus congestions.

- **Eucalyptus tea** will help clear out congested lungs and sinuses, and it can also help relieve the pain and stiffness associated with arthritis.

- **Olive oil** will reduce the risk of developing cardiovascular disease.

- **Peppermint** is a delicious herb that will help relieve gas and bloating, chronic indigestion, headaches, and muscle aches.

- **Pumpkin seeds** have compounds that will help to heal skin irritations.

- **Rosemary** can be used to season your food or made into tea. Either way, it will help relieve arthritis pain and muscle aches.

- **Sage** used in your recipes will help with your digestive issues, and if you make it into tea, it will help relieve fevers and symptoms of the common cold.

- **Sesame** will help your body to have lower blood pressure and lower bad cholesterol.

- **Thyme** will make your food taste great while helping calm your coughing or easing your lung congestion.

- **Turmeric** has long been known to relieve inflammation.

You can easily add more herbs to your daily diet so that the foods that you eat will help heal your body while making your food taste wonderful. Every time that you go to the grocery store, you should check out one or two new herbs that you have not tried before. When you make it a habit to buy herbs regularly, you will be creating the habit of using them in your recipes regularly. You might even want to try your hand at growing an herb garden, even if it is just a few pots of herbs sitting in the window of your kitchen. Even someone who lives in an apartment can find space to grow a few herbs. And if the fresh herbs are right there where you are cooking, you will be more likely to use them regularly. Fresh herbs will have more compounds that will make your food taste good while they heal your body.

If you buy your herbs in bulk, you may find that you will save time and money in preparing them. When you buy the herbs, plan to prepare them all at the same time. If you are trying to chop the herb and it won't easily chop, it might not be dry enough. It is an easy matter to save leftover herbs and extra herbs. One excellent way to store herbs is to freeze them into ice cubes. This method will serve two purposes. It will give you a way to store the herb safely, and it will give you frozen herbs in ice cubes to add to your morning smoothies.

Herbs help promote a relaxing environment, so your body will support your mental, emotional, and physical rejuvenation and stability. Herbs will set the foundation to heal illnesses and diseases and prevent chronic diseases from ever developing. Herbs can be used in many different combinations to give the same body area assistance or fight the same condition. Herbs can assist with the health of a wide array of conditions and can be beneficial to several organs all at once. That is good because no organ in your body works by itself; all of them are interconnected somehow. When you combine herbs with setting a target at a specific illness or a particular area of the body, it will increase the herb's overall effectiveness in its ability to heal your body. Herbs are an important part of the Alkaline Diet.

When Should I Consume the Revitalizing Herbs?

The best time to consume the revitalizing herbs is the next day after you finish your cleanse. For instance, if you fast for 14days, on the 15day, you should start consuming your revitalizing herbs.

What Are the Things That I Shouldn't Forget?

- Drink at least a gallon of spring water daily.

- Once you are done with your detox /cleanse, eat foods only on Dr. Sebi's nutritional guide.

- Consume the revitalizing herbs, including Irish Sea moss and sarsaparilla root.

- Ensure you do an intra-cellular cleanse once per year for at least 7days if you consume only an alkaline diet from Dr. Sebi's nutritional guide. Still, if you are not, you should always do an intra-cellular cleansing after every three months.

Please note that consuming acidic food can only put your body at the risk of relapsing.

Keeping the body healthy

Maintaining a Healthy Weight

Maintaining a healthy weight is important for renal patients as frequent weight changes may further damage your kidneys and harm your health. You need to make sure that you are not overeating to make up because you are missing out on certain types of meals as you are restricted from some food groups that may also harm your condition and damage your renal functions. The best way of maintaining a healthy weight is to eat regularly and try having smaller meal portions with fewer calories while taking all the nutrients you need. Follow up with tips we have previously listed for healthier weight maintenance, which means that you should avoid extra fat, sugar, and processed foods for the best results. Eating regularly and establishing a routine with your meals is also recommended. When it comes to food preparation, as mentioned earlier in the book, use cooking techniques that originally require less oil and fat for preparation. Your diet may be diverse; however, you need to take care of portions and avoid responding to food cravings and eating more than your body needs.

Watch Your Calorie Intake

Calories should be watched closely in terms of avoiding consuming empty calories. This kind can give you the energy your body needs, but that won't offer the essential nutrients that your body needs. Empty calories are usually found in sweets, sugary beverages, and snacks. Avoid munching on snacks and sweets and find healthier alternatives in fruit and vegetables. These food groups will provide you with all essential nutrients and have fewer calories than processed food with added sugar or added sodium.

Don't Take Weight Supplements

Maintaining a healthy weight is important for your health and will help you live a normal life even when your renal system is giving you a hard time; however, you should never take an alternative in a shortcut, meaning that you shouldn't rely on weight supplements and weight loss products for helping you lose or maintain your weight. Weight supplements may impose more threat to your health by adding more toxins and waste to your organism.

No Over-the-Counter Pills and Medications

Common pain killers usually taken and bought over the counter and without a prescription and used to diminish or relieve pain, and anti-inflammatory drugs raise the risk of getting a kidney's disease or have the kidney's condition worsened when taken regularly. Avoid taking pain killers unless prescribed by your doctor otherwise. If in pain, talk to your physician or a doctor specialist about which medications are safe for you. Avoid taking any type of medicines and pills that are no9t specifically prescribed for you and your doctor. Your condition will most certainly worsen as you will be placing extra pressure on your kidneys due to these medications' consumption.

Avoid Sweets and Sugar-packed Goods

Patients with diabetes represent a risk group for getting chronic kidney diseases as well. In contrast, patients with kidney conditions may worsen with the frequent consumption of sugar and processed foods with added sugar. Just as we recommend cutting on your salt consumption to avoid having an increased sodium level in your body and further complications caused by redundant sodium, it is likewise recommended to cut on your sugar intake. Sugar may cause diabetes if taken regularly and in large quantities and should be avoided. You may use fruit as a way healthier alternative but try to avoid high-potassium foods such as bananas.

Get Plenty of Sleep

Sleep deprivation may cause all kinds of health conditions that cause further damage to the body. That's because we use sleep to help our cells renew, and our bodies recover. Whenever we don't get enough sleep, we get tired, feel fatigued, our blood pressure is fluctuating, we lose focus, and we are often unable to perform daily tasks we normally do. Not getting the sleep you need will also make your body more prone to all kinds of disease and illness, while it will make your entire body feel alarmed and stressed, which should further have a devastating effect on your renal health. Make sure to address your body's needs and get as much sleep as you need.

Eat Healthy

Eating healthy should be the centerpiece of your new lifestyle as healthy food improves health and has numerous benefits for our body and mind. When eating unhealthy food in the long run, we introduce our body to lots of waste that our organism doesn't need, which is where the role of kidneys and our renal functions comes as crucial for our well-being. In cases where renal function is weak, slow, or failing in performance, waste introduced through an unhealthy diet causes various damage to the body. Furthermore, it brings more damage to the kidneys and renal system, creating a vicious circle where your health condition is only getting worse. Make sure to cut on fast food and snacks, junk food, processed food, sweets, and food packed with salt and additives. Focus on fresh groceries and healthily prepared food.

Check Your Blood Pressure

Blood pressure is the cause of many serious health conditions, and it also represents one of the main causes and symptoms of renal diseases. High blood pressure causes kidney damage and may harm your cardiovascular health, and cause a heart attack. In case you have high blood pressure, you should cut on your sodium intake. At the same time, kidney patients are advised to lower their sodium intake at all costs to prevent increased blood pressure that is more likely to be triggered by salt intake and consumption of bad fat and highly processed foods. Instead of salt, try using garlic and lemon for most of your meals. While garlic holds anti-inflammatory properties and acts benevolently on our immune system, garlic is also said to lower your blood pressure. Ensure that you check your blood pressure with your doctor regularly to avoid further complications and more damage to your kidneys.

Check Your Blood Sugar

As mentioned earlier, kidney disease can even be triggered by diabetes. In cases where patients develop diabetes due to an improper diet or/and genetic predispositions, kidney disease's overall condition is set to worsen. That is why we recommend cutting on sugary treats and beverages, added sugar, and processed foods. Preparing your food by yourself to follow up on the amounts of sugar present in your everyday diet.

Quit Smoking!

Smoking may cause all kinds of cancer, stroke, heart attack, and cardiovascular diseases, and it also increases the chances of getting kidney cancer. Patients who had already been diagnosed with a kidney disease should stop smoking as inhaling cigarette smoke may cause further damage to the kidneys because smoking slows down the flow of blood that runs through the kidneys, disabling these vital organs from performing functions that are crucial for your health.

Cut Your Meat Meals

Meat is packed with protein, and your kidneys are set to eject the leftover waste produced when our organism processes the protein, and our muscles take what they need from nutrients introduced with meat. Meat is delicious and nutritious, yes; however, too much meat is surely set to mess with your health and will place more pressure on your kidneys. Processed protein creates waste that your body needs to get rid of; as mentioned before, this waste is called urea and creatinine, and our body ejects it with the help of kidneys and through urine that way keeping us healthy and our body free of waste. To improve your renal health, you may seek meat substitution in salmon or start eating meat moderately and in smaller portions. The general recommendation would be twice to three times a week, once a day for meat portions, while you should also make sure to cook your meat with less oil and no fat added. Make sure to choose meat pieces that have less fat and more lean meat. Cook or slow cook your meat with herbs and spices instead of frying your meat and adding salt.

No Alcohol

Drinking is proven to have devastating effects on kidneys even at people who haven't been diagnosed with a form of kidney disease, as frequent and excess alcohol consumption increases the risk of getting a type of chronic kidney disease and brings extended damage to an already damaged renal system. Stay away from alcohol, even if you feel tempted. Alcohol is another form of liquid that your kidneys need to process and take care of, alongside introducing toxins to your body that may cause inflammation. Sugary alcohol beverages additionally contribute to weight gain, which could consequently bring more damage to your kidneys.

Dietary Choices for a Healthier Lifestyle

Your diet and lifestyle choices can make a huge difference to your daily life, the symptoms you experience, and the rate at which this develops in the early stages of kidney disease. Changes can even prevent your kidneys from deteriorating, give you more energy, help you maintain a healthy weight, and prevent illnesses and infections.

Overall, there are four main elements that you should be focusing on within your diet: phosphorous, potassium, sodium, and protein intake should be limited, and by making these changes in the early stages of the disease, you may even be able to prevent a far stricter diet in the later stages of the disease.

Unfortunately, many of us consume the diet in the US, and other western countries is not beneficial to our health. Nutritionists have termed the 'Standard American Diet' is unhealthy in many different respects: while including high levels of saturated fats, processed foods, and animal fats, it is also light on complex carbohydrates, fiber, fruits, and vegetables. All of this leads to a dramatically increased chance of stroke, heart disease, obesity, cancer, and, of course, kidney disease.

One of the main issues in this diet is processed food, when chemicals have been added to food to preserve and make it readily available to the consumer. In addition to these chemicals, processed foods include upwards of four times as much sugar as their natural counterparts. Excessive sugar levels increase the risk of type 2 diabetes, raise cholesterol levels, and creates a build-up of fat around the liver. As the liver works alongside the kidneys to remove toxins from the body, it is clear how these dietary choices can drastically increase kidney disease risk.

Always consult your doctor and nutritionist because it is the best thing to devise a meal plan specifically suited to your needs and the stage of the disease you are in. It is also important that you monitor and control your calorie intake as a loss of appetite is commonly experienced as a side effect of the disease. Therefore weight loss needs to be carefully monitored.

- **Carbohydrates and Fiber:** Although carbohydrates may be difficult to process at later stages of kidney disease, they provide a vital energy source that can combat lethargy feelings. As a low protein diet is recommended, carbohydrates can also help to replace calories. Some carbohydrates are also sources of fiber. It is recommended that you eat at least 25 grams of fiber per day, even when suffering from stage 5 kidney disease and undergoing dialysis. You may become frustrated when trying to count your fiber levels. Many high fibrous foods are also high in potassium, phosphorous, and fluid (all restricted). The food lists are a useful starting point for ingredients and their various nutritional values.

- **Fats:** Fats often get a bad reputation as we don't distinguish between healthy and unhealthy fats. Polyunsaturated and monounsaturated fats are healthy when consumed in moderation, whereas trans fats and saturated fats should be avoided.

- **Protein:** Although bodybuilders usually come to mind when we think of protein, it is an essential component of our diets and vital for repairing tissues, keeping infections at bay, and, of course, building muscle, even in the most exercise-phobic of us! Suppose you have chronic kidney disease in the first few stages. In that case, it is usually advised to consume protein for up to 15% of your daily diet, with carbohydrates and fats making up 85%, the same amount recommended for an average adult's daily intake. At stage 4, this recommendation usually decreases to only 10% protein. During stage 5, and if you are on dialysis, the dialysis will filter out the waste toxins from your body and protein; therefore, you must include protein as part of your diet. Please note that you must follow your doctor's advice on how much protein you should be consuming at each stage, as it depends on various factors such as your height, weight, and which stage of the disease you have. Always consult a professional for individual guidance before making any changes to your diet.

- **Phosphorus and Calcium:** Phosphates are salt compounds that include salt and other minerals; they work, as it does calcium, to strengthen and keep our bones healthy. Our kidneys usually remove extra phosphorous in the blood, but kidney disease will prevent this process from functioning as it should. Unfortunately, it's not as simple as just removing all phosphates from your diet as they are pretty much in most foods, but we can look out for those high in phosphorous. A list of foods and identifies whether they are low, medium, or high in phosphorous. You should typically stay away from processed foods as these often contain additives. Too much phosphorus can also lead to a calcium deficit, which can, in turn, lead to the extreme bouts of itchiness that many chronic kidney disease sufferers report. If low calcium levels persist, this can lead to further pain, a general weakening of the bones, and even bone disease. It might be that your doctor will recommend taking a calcium supplement if your phosphorus levels remain too high. After this, medicines known as phosphorous binders may be required but always consult a professional.

- **Fluids:** As the kidneys start to decrease in functionality, waste toxins and excess liquids are not removed from the body as they should be. That may lead to your doctor recommending you limit the liquids you consume. Thas is more likely during the later stages of kidney disease, and you should consult a professional for specific advice.

- **Potassium:** This is a mineral that has an essential role in keeping your heart healthy and regulating water levels in the body. Again, this is another mineral that is usually removed when in excess through the kidney filtration system. Too much of one particular mineral is problematic as the kidneys cannot remove it in the way they can when they are completely healthy. Still, extremely low levels are also harmful. Potassium is commonly found in many fruits and vegetables—stick with watermelon, tangerines, pineapple, berries, apples, cherries, pears, grapes, and peaches as low potassium fruits.

- **Iron:** Anyone whose chronic kidney disease has resulted in anemia will need extra iron in their diet. Options high in iron include iron-fortified cereals, kidney beans, lima beans, chicken, pork, beef, and liver. As some iron-rich sources may conflict with other dietary considerations such as protein, ensure you find out from your doctor which sources of iron you can have.

7 Worst Foods for your Health

1) Alcohol
2) Soy
3) Eggs
4) Dairy
5) Sweetened Juices
6) Coffee
7) Any kind of Meat

10 Important Alkaline Fruits and Vegetables that Fit the Alkaline Diet

1) Cucumber
2) Onions
3) Zucchini
4) Avocado
5) Lettuce

6) Elderberries
7) Seeded grapes
8) Mango
9) Papaya
10) Tamarind

Manage your Stress During Kidney Failure

When you are suffering from kidney failure, it's normal to be stressed out all the time. It might lead you to skip meals or even forgetting your medication, which might affect your health even more.

But you need to understand that life is full of hurdles and setbacks, and you really can't let them hold you back.

In that light, here are six tips to help you keep your stress under control:

Make sure to take some time just to relax and unwind. Try to practice deep breathing, visualization, meditation, or even muscle relaxation. All of these will help you to stay calm and keep your body healthy.

Try to accept the things that are not under your control, and you can't change. Trying to enforce a change on something that is not within your reach will only make things worse for you. Better advice is to look for better ways of handling the situation instead of trying to change it.

Don't pressure yourself; try to be good to yourself and don't expect much. You are a human being, after all, right? You can make mistakes, so accept that. Just try your best.

And lastly, always try to maintain a positive attitude. Even when things go completely wrong, try to see the good instead of the bad and focus on that. Try to find things in all phases of your life that make you happy and that you appreciate, such as your friends, work, health, and family, for example. You have no idea how much help a simple change of perspective can bring.

Keep yourself hydrated

You should always make sure that you are sufficiently hydrated, but you shouldn't overdo this. No studies have shown that over-hydration is good for enhancing the performance of your kidneys. It is good to drink sufficient water, and you can drink around four to six glasses of water per day. Consuming more water than this wouldn't help your kidneys perform better. It would just increase the stress on your kidneys.

Read the labels carefully

The next time you go shopping for groceries, make sure you carefully read the labels on food products. Read the nutritional chart that's printed on the cover, and if you don't recognize anything on it, it's better if you don't pick it up. You need to be very careful about the food products you consume when on a renal failure diet.

Accept Practical and Emotional Support

If you have a network of encouraging you, it is advantageous for your health, mostly emotional encouragement or support. Research conducted has put side by side individuals who had the most and smallest amount of social support. It was recorded that those who had the most social support had a much better quality of healthy life and lived longer.

Below are some recommended ideas for building a support system:

- Request for assistance or for someone who can listen. Individuals, in most cases, want to assist but do not know how to go about it. Therefore, you will have to be precise and state your request.

- Enter into a support group. Sharing with other people who have related experiences might assist you to cope.

- Encourage others; It will form a healthy cycle of giving and receiving.

Avoid Environmental Toxins

Reduce your exposure to environmental toxins that can raise your chances of having cancer and other deadly diseases, including asbestos, formaldehyde, tobacco smoke, styrene (seen in Styrofoam), and tetrachloroethylene (perchloroethylene).

Prepare Your Meals

The best way of knowing what you are consuming to the tiniest detail is to prepare your food by yourself; you may love take-outs and nights when you have your dinner out but try to prepare most of your food by yourself, including your snacks. When making your meals, make sure that the food you are using is mostly fresh and low in sodium, potassium, and low concentrations of other nutrients that can be harmful to your renal health. Try to take your lunch from home when going to work instead of eating in a cafeteria or a restaurant. Focus on preparing meals by boiling, steaming, slow cooking, or baking instead of frying techniques.

No Added Salt and Processed Foods

Besides encouraging more fresh groceries with low-sodium and low-potassium concentrations, we also encourage you to avoid adding salt to your meals and follow up with food labels to ensure that you are not consuming food with high concentrations sodium as well as potassium. Processed foods such as processed meat, boxed and packaged goods, snacks, junk food and fast food, sweets and cookies, candy, and similar sugary treats are bad for you in general, and with added salt may additionally harm our kidneys and slow down your renal functions, that way damaging your kidneys as these vital organs are not able to process and level all the sodium in your body with the presence of chronic kidney disease.

Watch for Your Potassium Intake

Follow up with the grocery list we have made on foods that are normally low in potassium concentrations so that your body may receive the quantity of this vital mineral it needs without struggling with excess waste. Be aware that some low-sodium products may have increased concentrations of potassium. Consult your doctor on potassium and discuss the average amount of potassium you may have on a weekly and daily basis with your condition.

Be Active and Exercise

Being active and exercising is important for everyone as your body needs activity to burn calories that you are introducing to your body with every meal. Physical activity also encourages serotonin production – the happiness hormone – which makes you feel motivated and refreshed once healthy physical activity becomes a part of your routine. Physical condition is great for your health and should help you battle issues you are having with your renal health. Make sure not to overestimate yourself or underestimate the effects of activity and exercising.

Common forms of exercise include:

- Stair climbing
- Tai Chi
- Stretching
- Yoga
- Cycling
- Walking
- Swimming

To perform these normal workouts, you don't have to join a gym or even buy any sort of expensive equipment! You can simply take a walk around your streets, do yoga at home, and so on.

Just make sure to consult with your doctor to determine which exercise is suitable for you and adjust it to your dialysis routine. If you were already consuming healthy foods, it would also make sense if you were exercising regularly because regular physical activity will prevent weight gain and regulate your blood pressure. But you should be careful about the amount of time you exercise or how much you exercise, especially if you aren't acclimatized to exercising. Don't overexert yourself if you are just getting started because this would increase your kidneys' pressure and break down your muscles.

Seek treatment for hypertension

The pressure is now considered the leading cause of chronic renal failure. According to nephrologist Nestor Scho, professor at Unifesp, the increase in blood pressure damages the kidneys' blood vessels and may cause hypertensive nephropathy. "This way, the organ becomes overloaded, and little by little loses its filtering capacity," he explains. Taking care of hypertension is essential even when it is not the cause of chronic renal failure, as it becomes even more important in the advanced stage of the disease.

Control of diabetes

"Diabetes is the second leading cause of chronic renal failure," says nephrologist Lucio Roberto Moura of Hospital Israelita Albert Einstein. That is because the disease triggers the so-called 'diabetic nephropathy', a change in kidney vessels that leads to a protein loss in the urine. Also, diabetes favors atherosclerosis, forming plaque fat in the arteries that hinders the kidneys' filtration work. Over time, more and more toxic substances are trapped in the body, leading to death. Therefore, one way to detect the problem is to do urine tests to determine if the protein is being eliminated. Those already diagnosed with diabetes need to be more aware of their kidney health.

If you want to know more about the topic of Diabetes and Hypertension and how you can treat them, check out my book:

" Dr.Sebi Diet: Your Essential Guide to Reversing Diabetes and High Blood Pressure By Living the Dr.Sebi Lifestyle".

Chapter 11: Supplements

The very best approach to acquire the critical substances you desire (minerals, vitamins, essential fatty acids, fats -- the list continues on and on) is via a balanced, healthful, nutritional supplement (one which is 100 percent natural if possible). However, the truth is that several individuals have quite a difficult time eating enough of the ideal sorts of foods to acquire the materials they require in the right amounts. That is why it is highly suggested that you carefully think about using nutritional supplements to improve the quantities of crucial stuff your body needs to work at its best.

It might appear overwhelming to consider carrying ten (or more) distinct supplements daily but remember that doing this could be a true advantage to your body and head. Additionally, it might allow you to stay longer and much healthier. Nevertheless, suppose you are aware that you are getting a fantastic amount of a few of these chemicals in your diet plan. You are interested in maintaining the number of supplements you are taking comparatively low. In that case, you can correct your nutritional regimen so. For example, if you consume lots of fatty, cold-water fish, you might not have to supplement using omega-3 fatty acids. Consider your daily diet and nutritional supplement in a proper method to ensure you're giving your body exactly what it requires.

Here is one important note to remember while you're considering nutritional supplements: Your daily recommended allowances for vitamins, minerals, nutritional supplements, and other chemicals that you see on food labels do not indicate a great deal. These tips show you the minimum quantities necessary for the body to keep working properly. However, they do not let you know what amounts you will need for the body to go beyond that foundation level.

Multivitamin

Some people today choose a once-a-day multivitamin. While that is better than simply taking nothing in any way, the tablet likely does not include large enough dosages of all the vitamins you want. How can I know? Suppose a once-a-day vitamin comprised adequately substantial doses of 14 essential vitamins. In that case, it might need to be as large as a golf club. The majority of the multivitamins offering comprehensive vitamin policy ask that you take a few pills every day. Four capsules or tablets per day is a fairly typical number.

A variety of great brands and moderately priced options can be found. You would like to locate an organization that does third party analysis. Most of their better products aren't offered across the counter. They have to be bought via an undercover doctor or a drugstore involved in natural wellbeing. Guarantee that the multivitamin you select includes a great calcium source and be certain it functions as calcium hydroxylapatite rather than calcium carbonate. You do not automatically realize the differences between both; simply ensure your multivitamin involves the former rather than the latter.

Multimineral

In general, you will need to provide your system using 16 distinct nutritional supplements if you would like it to perform at an optimum level.

Multimineral nutritional supplements are simple to discover. In several instances, you can discover multivitamin/multi-mineral combination nutritional supplements. These options can be challenging, and you have to be certain if you decide to go that path; you purchase an option that comprises all 14 vitamins and all 16 nutritional supplements. (That is rather a good deal!)

If you are picking a multi-mineral supplement, then go with one which features chelated minerals. I will spare you all of the full details of this procedure, which produces chelated minerals. But remember that you are likely paying for nutritional supplements that wind up on your bathroom rather than on your own body's major systems unless you are getting chelated minerals.

Do not choose a multi-mineral supplement that arrives out of a clay resource. These goods aren't chelated, plus they feature tin, silver, and nickel. Sometimes they even record lead as a component!

Omega-3 Fatty Acids

You have probably read or heard about omega-3 fatty acids in the news lately. The significance of this essential fatty acid was getting a great deal of press and great reason. It is one of these substances your body needs to endure and flourish. Despite all of the wonderfully intricate chemical processes that your own body can perform, it cannot fabricate omega-3 fatty acids.

The best dietary source of omega-3s is beef. Fish is another great resource. You ought to consume fish as part of a proper diet; however, unless you are eating wild Alaskan salmon, or even among those other few kinds of fish which do not commonly contain elevated levels of mercury, it is likely that you're becoming an extremely salty dose of toxins with your omega-3 fatty acids.

To stay clear of germs but get your omega-3 supplement, use liquid fish oil or even some capsule or soft gel. Take 1 g twice per day to get what you want.

Resveratrol

Resveratrol is a highly effective antioxidant, and I recommend that everybody get a dose of this every day. Resveratrol has generated a higher profile as a Harvard Medical School case study. A couple of years back, a fairly dramatic gain in mice's health and lifespan was revealed after they were given resveratrol. Should you read up about this particular antioxidant, you're likely to see it is in red wine, which is the reality. However, suppose you wished to receive an important dose of resveratrol from red wine. In that case, you'd need to glug a couple of hundred bottles of the material daily, which will kill you before you have to enjoy the advantages of resveratrol.

The fantastic thing is you can purchase resveratrol supplements in many health food shops and any vitamin store, either in person or on the internet. You will find it labeled either as resveratrol or red wine extract. I suggest getting 30 mg every day that ought to be somewhat simple, given the width of nutritional supplement options available in the industry.

Vitamin C

If you choose a fantastic multivitamin, you will likely get a fantastic amount of vitamin C every day. But do not believe for a moment you are getting all your body should truly have the ability to work on a full degree.

I suggest carrying a 1,000-milligram vitamin C supplement two times every day. I know that seems like a great deal, but if you've read about it, you understand why I believe very strongly that vitamin C is a massive blessing for your great health. Though it's within plenty of vegetables and fruits, it may continue to be hard to get enough of the things on your diet plan. Hundreds (maybe thousands) of vitamin C supplement options are available, so do some research and speak with your naturopathic physician to discover which ones are ideal for you.

If you are fighting a disease, take 8,000 mg of vitamin C daily rather than the normal 2,000 mg.

Vitamin B Complex

The term vitamin B complex describes all of the B vitamins: B1, B2, B3, B5, B6, B7, B9, and B12. A number of the B vitamins also have several other widely used titles – riboflavin and niacin are just two great examples.

The assortment of important features the vitamin B complex performs on the human body is shocking, and I would not even try to cover all of the details. Just know that if you want to be healthy and live a long, comfy lifestyle, you had better concentrate on getting lots of B vitamins.

It's a fantastic idea to have a vitamin B complex supplement as well as a multivitamin daily. You'll discover such a supplement that can provide you exactly what you need in just one dose every day.

Magnesium

Several strong studies performed over the past couple of years have demonstrated powerful connections between elevated levels of magnesium intake and cardiovascular disease avoidance. Individuals who get lots of calcium – within their diets and during supplementing – normally possess a reduced heart disease risk. Additionally, magnesium is also involved in approximately 300 different biochemical reactions that happen within your own body, which means that you may see why it is a fantastic idea to be certain that you're getting enough. To be sure, have a supplement which provides you 600 mg each day.

Sulforaphane

Not everybody has heard of sulforaphane, and that is too bad. It has been making headlines on a fairly regular basis recently, and everybody ought to be carrying it as a nutritional supplement regularly.

Recent studies have suggested that sulforaphane will help thwart some sorts of cancer and may slow tumor growth. Additional studies reveal that sulforaphane lessens the quantity of H. pylori bacteria from the gut, which triggers stomach lining inflammation and nausea. If those are not good reasons to choose sulforaphane every day, I do not understand what exactly they are.

You're able to get sulforaphane in supplement form in 2 manners: carrot seed infusion or plain sulforaphane. If you go for the latter, then take 500 mg daily. In case the prior is the favorite sulforaphane nutritional supplement, attempt to receive 30 mg daily.

Vitamin E

Along with vitamin C and vitamin B complex, vitamin E is something that will almost surely be included in your multivitamin routine but likely not in large enough quantities. You'll be able to see continuing health benefits of supplementing with vitamin E around 800 mg every day, and therefore don't be reluctant to take that much.

What are a few of the health advantages of taking extra vitamin E? To begin with, vitamin E has strong antioxidant effects. But vitamin E does several other fantastic things for the body, too, from boosting your immune system to maintaining blood vessels at tiptop form.

Do yourself massive favor, and do not scrimp on the vitamin E.

Alpha-Lipoic Acid (ALA)

You will frequently see the lipoic acid known as ALA. It is a top-notch antioxidant that helps your body fight infection and retains your cells working at a higher level.

Choose an ALA nutritional supplement and locate a capsule type that produces about 800 mg every day. That amount was demonstrated to provide many health benefits with no overpowering or side-effects within the human body. It's possible to locate ALA supplements in any fantastic health food shop and the regional vitamin retailer.

Conclusion

We encourage you to return to our guidebook any time you are in doubt or whenever you would like to get back to useful tips on how to live a healthier life with damaged renal functions and chronic kidney disease. The state of your renal function defines how well your organism and your body are functioning; however, as explained in the book, your health should see crucial improvements with the change of your everyday diet.

Make sure always to check your labels when shopping for groceries and take care that the meals you are preparing are made ready following the low-potassium and low-sodium diet for best results and remember that healthy habits make a healthy life.

Patients who struggle with kidney health issues, going through kidney dialysis, and having renal impairments need to go through medical treatment and change their eating habits and lifestyle to make the situation better. Much research has been done on this, and the conclusion is that food has a lot to do with how your kidney functions and its overall health.

The first thing to changing your lifestyle is knowing how your kidney functions and how different foods can trigger different kidney function reactions. Certain nutrients affect your kidney directly. Nutrients like sodium, protein, phosphate, and potassium are the risky ones. You do not have to omit them altogether from your diet, but you need to limit or minimize their intake as much as possible. You cannot leave out essential nutrients like protein from your diet, but you need to count how much protein you are having per day. It is essential to keep balance in your muscles and maintaining a good functioning kidney.

At the point when you eat flippantly and fill your body with toxins, either from nourishment, drinks (liquor or alcohol, for instance) or even from the air you inhale (free radicals are in the sun and move through your skin, through dirty air, and numerous food sources contain them). In general, your body will convert numerous things that appear to be benign until your body's organs convert them into things like formaldehyde because of a synthetic response and transforming phase.

A profound change in kidney patients is measuring how much fluid they are drinking. Too much water or any other form of liquid can disrupt their function. How much fluid you can consume depends on your kidney's condition. Most people assign separate bottles to measure how much they have drunk and how much more they can drink throughout the day.

Like all other body parts, human kidneys also need much care and attention to work effectively. It takes a few simple and consistent measures to keep them healthy. Remember that no medicine can guarantee good health, but only a better lifestyle can do so.

Since the early signs of kidney disease are hardly detectable, it is important to keep track of the changes you witness in your body. Even the frequency of urination and loss of appetite are good enough reasons to be cautious and concerning. Indeed, only a health expert can accurately diagnose the disease, but personal care and attention to minor changes are of key importance to CKD.

Made in the USA
Coppell, TX
14 July 2021